A User Manual for Living Healthy

CARE
FOR YOUR
HEALTH

DR BISWAJIT MOHAPATRA, MS

Consultant Laparoscopic Surgeon,
NLP Health Motivator, Speaker. Odisha, India
9437042490.
bmdoc1@gmail.com

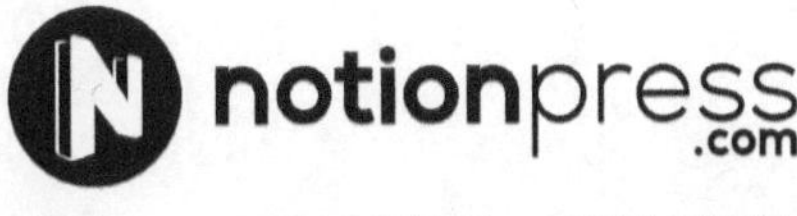

Notion Press

Old No. 38, New No. 6
McNichols Road, Chetpet
Chennai - 600 031

First Published by Notion Press 2019
Copyright © Biswajit Mohapatra 2019
All Rights Reserved.

ISBN 978-1-64546-503-4

Contents

CHAPTER I

Introduction

"Taking full responsibility for a healthy life is the beginning of a successful journey on the life's path".

Author

It is a calling from the higher self, that I am writing this book. As far as I can go back to my early years, I vividly remember the Hospital where my father was working as a pharmacist. Ispat General Hospital is my childhood inspiration, which still stands tall in front of me, as an icon of healthcare to the people of this part of the country. I have seen the healthcare scenario changing over four decades. I have seen it as a child, as a son of a pharmacist, as a medical officer of a small industry to as a consultant in practice. I have also seen my own perception changing over the years from a compassionate doctor to a passionate health activist. I am a witness to the approach of modern medicine changing from caring to managing patients.

When I think of my last 25 years of surgical practice, I feel proud to be a part of a profession, which has a clear understanding about the value of life. How I have managed thousands of critically ill patients with minimum resources and send most of them home happy, is a subject of discussion. It is time now, after 25 years to recollect those periods and to acknowledge the help of God for my successful career till date. I always give credit of my success to this amazing body created by God, with so much miraculous healing power. I operate but He cures. This body has all the power to heal, and we doctors take advantage of this power to treat people

This book is just a recollection of my experience and about the possibility of a disease free world. It is a big dream, but not impossible. My association with both the diseases and diseased persons always remind me of a saying from old literature, "future of medicine will be not on the research molecules but will depend on how good we are in preventing diseases". Whenever I see a pathient coming to me with pain and agony, I always ask myself, could the person have prevented this? Most of the time an answer echoes inside my heart ... Yes.

As years passed by, my conviction on this inner voice started getting bigger and bigger. 10 years back I started on this mission of educating and informing the general mass on cancer prevention. I started visiting places and groups where the incident of cancer was more. After about a year, when I analyzed my work and its impact on the people, I was shaken. The results were a big failure and were wastage of time. The reason being, the people whom I targeted were not in need of my preaching but they were in need of some help in terms of finance or medications. As the old saying goes nothing flows from below upwards, information always percolates from above to below.

With that realization, I changed my strategy, and decided to spread the awareness among the responsible and educated mass. As my experience to educate the mass increased, I noticed a very unusual trend in my audience. The more I started talking about disease prevention, the more fearful my patients become. Their anxiety level increased to a higher level and most of them started feeling as a victim of the disease. I came across a book on laws of attraction this time. According to the law of attraction, the more we think about diseases, the more we attract those diseases. Mrs. D was one of those patients, who changed my perception totally.

I met Mrs. D one morning, in my OPD. She was referred to me for breast examination. Her history was vague. One of her friend was diagnosed with breast cancer. Since then she had a fear that, she is suffering from the same disease as her friend and consulted her gynaecologist two months back. The gynaecologist could not find any lump, so she sends her home after a brief counselling. Mrs. D visited twice more to the Gynecologist, before she referred Mrs. D to me for further evaluation. This woman had attended one of my awareness programs before coming to me. When I examined Mrs. D, there was no lump in her breast. She went on telling me all the signs and symptoms of breast cancer. After a proper examination, I wrote down few diagnostic tests to confirm, whether there is any evidence of tumour in her breast or not.

Next day morning she arrived with her reports and all were normal. With that after a good counselling, I taught her the breast self-examination and sent her home with a few vitamins. The story did not end there; she again dropped in to my cabin, exactly one month after my first appointment. Now she was very much sure of a small tumour on that spot, where she had shown me last time. This time also I could not find any abnormality and sent her home with assurance and anxiolytics. I thought she would be all right, but I was wrong. She dropped in again after two months with the same complain and asked me to redo all the tests. This time I asked her for a FNAC (fine needle aspiration cytology) from the site she was showing me, for her satisfaction. She readily agreed and I took little fluid, from the area of breast she was showing me and asked her to see me after two days.

I was surprised to get a call next day from our pathologist, asking me to send a bigger tissue sample from that area. According to him, the cytology looked normal, but he could find one or two suspicious cells. Therefore, he wanted to confirm it before giving a report. Then I immediately messaged her to meet me. Next day she arrived with her husband and I explained her situation and the need for a biopsy. They panicked and wanted to take her to a cancer institute for further confirmation, which I did and referred her to Tata memorial hospital, (TMH) Mumbai.

For the next few months, I did not receive any news from Mrs. D or from her husband. Then one morning Mr. D came to meet me and narrated her story. TMH doctors reviewed the slides and gave her a green signal that no cancer cell was found in that slide. There also she insisted for a biopsy, so the surgeon there decided to go for a frozen section biopsy. During operation on table, frozen section biopsy was done from the suspicious area. Unfortunately, that turned out as cancer.

They did a clearance of that area and the patient was put on chemo and radiation. Mr. D told me, her operating surgeon had thanked me for sending a patient so early to him, but I was convinced that, she manifested the cancer in her body during that period of constant belief of having a cancer in her breast. When I met her after a week, I found her in a peaceful state, as the fear of cancer was no more in her mind.

This incidence made me to think about the cancer awareness program. I have started asking myself a question that 'am I not creating more fear among people by educating them about the diseases'? For the first time I had doubt about my own programs. This was time I decided for a different approach. We can prevent all these diseases, if I can somehow motivate people to adopt a healthy lifestyle.

Soon I realized that it is a mammoth task to spread awareness about healthy living. The reason being, people who do not have time, even to think about their health. Health is the last priority among the majority. The other major factors, which I noticed was the belief system of the people that, consult doctors when you are ill. Many people dogmatically follow the advice of religious leaders and health food seller's advertisement influence others.

The most unfortunate part was the, great silence from doctors like us, who knows about the human body and mind but not ready to share it with patients. This has only helped to aggravate this situation.

I was very much convinced that only information is not enough to attract people to attend my talk, I had to motivate them to follow my talk. Therefore, for the first time I have started to coin the term health motivation, to woo them to listen to me. Instead of telling them the facts, I have started explaining them the space between the facts and narrating them the extraordinary stories of my patients, their journey on the healing path and the miracle of this human body. I made them visualize the power they posses and the power of self-love. Suddenly I found my audience and gradually I graduated from a Surgeon to a **Health Motivator**. Now it was my turn to get ready, deliver quality information to you all, and motivate the mass. It was a difficult task to structure the program, which could keep audience for hours to listen to me. This book, which I have written, is all about the way I have simplified the information and inculcated in a common person's mind.

CHAPTER II

Care for Your Health

"If we have to win over diseases, which are going to destroy the majority of population in near future, it's you and me, who has to do the groundwork. Be a part of the "Care for Your health" movement. "Prevention is the future of medicine"

Author

What Is CFYH

"Care for Your health' movement is a small step towards a big Health Revolution. When the whole world is looking for a solution of their diseases in the present modern medical system, this movement will spread light on the way we should live, so that we will not ever need the help of this Newtonian Health care system, where matter get priority over energy. As per new Biology, we all are energy vibrations and connected with each other and governed by universal consciousness. We are blessed with the power of recreating ourselves at any moment of time by simply changing our perception to our immediate environment. Our perception again depends on our belief system, which is the result of constant bombardment of certain information on our brain cells. This results in formation of a pattern of wiring in our brain. There is a saying, "neurons fire together, wire together". Therefore, our biology is directly under the influence of our belief system.

Today's "Health care system" is a misnomer. It should have been named "Disease care system", as this system takes care of our diseases, not our health. Health is a natural phenomenon, where as disease is an intrusion into the nature. With the world population increasing in an explosive manner, we are falling short of resources to manage the numbers. This has already created a fear all over the world. Future looks dangerous. However, we all have a hope, if we just twist the nomenclature "Health Care" system to "Care for Health" System. I could see the possibility of a new era of medicine, where every person will, take care of his/her health and follow certain rules, so that he will not fall ill. This requires a more aggressive approach then the present "Health Care" system. The rules here are simple but mandatory to follow. Hope I could put some light on this system of medicine through this book, so that people will be able to take decisions about themselves properly. This needs a change in our belief system,

To change our belief system, we have to rewire our brain cells by feeding it with newer information or knowledge. When we will be able to influence the general mass by empowering them with knowledge about themselves, through movement like "Care for Your Health", there is a hope for a healthy tomorrow. This will one day turn the mind of a common person from disease consciousness to health conscious.

Few days back I was invited to a conclave to speak on a topic, "Health Care at your Door Step". I pondered over the topic and tried to figure out, in what way it is possible. With the widening doctor patient ratio, increasing disease burden, increasing stress level, poor food habits, poverty and illiteracy, I found this topic is only for discussion. I chose to speak on the possibility of "Care for your Health" at door Step. It was widely acknowledged.

Health is our birthright, 95 percent of us are born healthy. Nevertheless, as our life progresses, our environment, our family, our education system, our eating habits, starts influencing us and we start forgetting our natural potentials, which is an integral part of the nature. This leads us to a state of disharmony with the nature and then the disease and illness sets in. Once we start focusing on our strength, we automatically become powerful to keep illness at bay. When we adopt "Care for Your Health", our inner self awaken, to help us to lead a life of peace, prosperity, and happiness. This is the time when every single cell of our body works in harmony with the nature and leads us to a state of pure health.

Maintaining a sound health takes less effort than restoring normalcy from a diseased state. In my 30 years in medical profession, I have rarely seen pious people like yogis and other religious gurus suffering from illness, as they follow certain rules to protect their body and mind, by regular meditation, exercise, and regular food habits in their lifetime.

I recently met one brahmakumari, who had cervical cancer, 20 years back. That was the time she chose to follow the spiritual path and dedicated her life for the service of higher self. She followed all those rituals regularly and her disease has not returned to her since then. In NLP [Neuro LingisticProgrammimg] we have a pre supposition, "if one can do it, anyone can do it". This book will emphasize on those rules in the subsequent chapters, so that readers will find it easier to follow.

"Care for Your Health" is not going to be limited to this book only. It is our responsibility to create a movement, through which we can share the secrets of living healthy to every person on this planet. This movement of health consciousness will prevent diseases largely. This is not a one man's job and needs millions of hands to materialize it. This can be possible by creating "CFYH Centre" at every place, where we can train people to keep themselves healthy. My dream is one day CFYH Centres will replace the existing Health Care Centres, which will educate the general mass about Health and happiness. Please do visit my website www.careforyourhealth.in and be a part of this movement.

Chapter III

Care for Your Cells

Our body is a wonderful creation of God. It has all the software pre installed, which can be used to reboot ourselves, whenever in need. Only you have to be literate enough to operate this machine, called human body.

Author

Why do you think it is necessary to make people understand about their biology? One of my friends asked me during the preparation for my presentation. He is a reputed medical practitioner in our city. I just asked him; do you ever pass on the information about the amazing power of our body to your patients? He was unable to answer my question immediately, so I narrated the following reason for this approach to him.

After doing my Masters in General Surgery, in 1995, I immediately joined as a senior residency program in my own collage. During these formative years as a surgeon, I only did operations and taught my juniors, the techniques of surgical procedures. By the time I left medical college and joined my practice at my hometown as a consultant, I graduated to become a perfect surgical artisan.

During the initial years of my practice, I was busy with my surgeries and I was getting wonderful results. The more surgeries I did, the more confident, I became. That was the time; I started noticing something unusual with the postoperative recovery of my patients. For the same surgeries, two patients used to get two different course of response. I started noticing the requirements of analgesics were different in different groups of patients. I witnessed events, which I could not explain by the conventional knowledge, which I had at that particular time. All these led me to think little bit laterally and I started looking for the alternate sources to get an explanation.

This was the time accidentally I came across the book "Biology of belief", written by Dr. Bruce Lipton. Suddenly I got the long awaited answers to my questions.

For the first time I realized, the new research in the field of cell biology has changed the concept of biology and now it is known as "New Biology". This has led me to go deep into the subject and update my knowledge base. Now it is my turn to pass on the newly learned concept to people and empower them with the knowledge to lead a healthy life.

This chapter is all about the God's marvellous creation..."Life". Unicellular organisms inhibited the earth for about 750 millions of years. 250 million years back, due to some environmental changes, they found it difficult to survive alone and started living in groups or colonies of thousands or more to cope up with the climatic change. With time, they could feel the evolutionary advantages of staying together. Their increased awareness to environment and shared workload lead them to become more organized, structured and disciplined. This is how the plants and other primitive multicellular organisms came into existence. With time, cells of these organisms started getting smarter and some of them trained themselves for certain specialized work and refused to do other functions. This resulted in formation of organ system, and the philosophy of distribution of labour came in to play. These specialized cells are our immune systems, our heart, our lungs, our nervous system, our excretory system etc. They operate intelligently-independently and interdependently through different messenger molecules.

To understand the human body, we have to understand the function of our own cells, which control our state of health and mind at each moment of our life. We are made up of 70 to 80 trillions of cells and every cell has a potential of a 'Miniature' human being. Our cells are the smallest living part of us. What we call as a human being is nothing but a community of trillions of obedient and sincere citizens living together peacefully. Every cell does the same function as we all human beings do. All the cells perform the functions of excretory system, respiratory system, digestive system, nervous, circulatory system etc. They are more intelligent than we are and follow the instructions of each other in a very synchronous way. According to Boyce Rensberger, each cell can take in information about its circumstances and respond to it purposefully. There are about 200 different type of cells found in our body, that make our tissues, organs and different systems. Our body is a universe by itself. Each cell has its own soul and intelligence. The instructions for all these different cells are hidden in its nucleus and written as codes on our DNA, which makes our chromosomes.

Each cell has the power to receive, analyze, and send information to the cells present far away through the matrix of the intercellular space. Cell biologists now call them "neuropeptide web," which is present in our cellular cytoskeleton. Our cytoskeleton is nothing but the structure on which 70 trillions of cells are woven by a network of proteins present outside the cell membrane, and give shapes and support to cells.

The way the cells communicate to each other is very complex but the recent research shows that, it is the physical twisting; bending and touching each other through constant change in shape initiate the cell-to-cell talk. Innumerable chemical, electromagnetic and informational messenger molecules, present all over the body known to us as neuropeptides, mostly induce this type of cell-to-cell talk.

This is where we have to understand the complex role played by "Psychoneuroimmunology". Candace Pert a Neuroscientist in her book "Molecules of emotion" writes we are not a 'Mind body' phenomenon but a 'body of minds', where the messenger molecules are constantly processing and responding, to the environment, to our thoughts, to our emotions and to the physical processes. This proves that our brain is not running the show from our head but from the intelligent molecules distributed all over our body. They are constantly sending and receiving signals to direct changes in cells, distributed throughout our body instantaneously. *So our cells are made of molecules, they communicate through molecules and responds to signals by changing existing molecules.*

Human Machinery

Our health or our disease status depends on the conditions of our cells. If our cells are in harmony with the nature, we are healthy and when there is an imbalance, disease sets in. If we ever get a chance to voyage inside the human body as a Cytonaut, we will be surprised to see the highly advanced human machinery inside our cells.

- We have millions of transformers to produce energy known as "Mitochondria".

- We have factories to produce the building blocks of our body "Ribosome".

- We have sophisticated computer chips present on the cell wall, known as "Receptors", which act as gateway to allow the information to get into the cell or allow the finished products to go out of the cells to its destination.

- We have millions of rechargeable batteries in our body known as ATP, which constantly produces, supplies and recharges itself for the next requirement of energy.

- We have worker molecules in our cells known as proteins, which provides the structure and do jobs like tissue formation, enzymes and hormones production.

- Our body has special garbage boxes known as lysosomes. This is where our dead cells and unwanted molecules gets destroyed and removed from the system.

- Home Office –nucleus acts as a well-advanced office with an up-to-date library, as it stores all the information for our body as codes in the DNA. It maintains it properly through our chromosomes.

- Our endomembrane (cytoplasm) system, works as a sophisticated manufacturing process and shipping plant. This acts as a post office of the cell. It is a system, which carries molecules to their destination.

Our body is just like a flowing river. The cells of our body are constantly getting replaced with new ones throughout our life. The gastric lining gets replaced once a week, the total skin gets replenished once a month. The skeleton of our body gets replaced every three months. Thus, a complete new human being is structured in three to five months.

Now the million-dollar question is what stops us to remain healthy forever, with such wonderful recreating mechanisms within us? Here we have to understand what makes our cells and how we can preserve it or keep ourselves healthy lifelong.

We are made up of four types of molecules, *proteins, carbohydrates and lipids and DNA.* Carbohydrates provide energy and structure to cells, lipids send signals and store energy and proteins are the main worker molecules of the cells as they are responsible for the main structure and for all important functions of the cells. Proteins control metabolism, transport, communications, structures and other aspect of cell functions. We are in fact a complex protein assembly of about more than 100000 different protein molecules to run this machine, called human body. Bruce Lipton in his book 'Biology of Belief' has mentioned, "Cells exploit the movement of these protein assembly machines to empower specific metabolic and behavioural function". We recycle tons of proteins every day due to death of about more than 300 millions of cells per minute and continue production of similar no of cells to replenish the dead cells. The blueprint to build different cell lies in the most famous *molecule of life* called DNA, which is the reproductive organ of cells. We have a gene for everything, from functional elements to behavioural and from metabolic elements to transportations. Our cell produces the required proteins when it receives signals for its need.

We believe that our DNA is responsible for everything what we are today and we are the victim of our DNA, as if our fate is predetermined. After the great "Human genome study", which lasted for about 12 years, we discovered that we have only 26000 genes, whereas the expected number was about 150000. Where were the missing genes? This finding led scientists working on cell biology to give a second thought. After further research they discovered that, a single gene can create 2000 or more variants of proteins depending on the different signals it receives from outside. This observation was the beginning of a new revolutionary field in biology called Epigenetic. This means control above genetics.

Epigenetic research has established that DNA is a blueprint and the information passed down through genes are not predetermined and not our destiny. Environmental influences including lifestyle, nutrition, stress, emotions can change those genes without changing their basic blueprints and can pass on to the future generations. The features of the code will manifest only when that particular code will express, copied by transcription RNA and sent to the factory (**Ribosome**) to produce the desired molecules. Almost all of us share the same genes in our body but we differ only by our expressive genes.

We perceive our environment through our five senses. We are constantly bombarded with information, which are filtered by our five senses and create our internal representations. Our internal representation directly affects our state of mind. Our emotions are the by-product of our state of mind and act as stimulus or signal for our cells to behave. Our thoughts, belief system, memory, experiences etc. play a great role in altering the state of our mind. Our state of mind has direct effect on our physiology, which leads to change in the chemical and molecular composition of our body. Our cells communicate through molecules and responds to signals by changing existing molecules or making new molecules.

The codes of our life are written in our DNA in chemical letters and are vulnerable to be changed under constant bombardment of altered signals. When there is a change in the code, it alters the gene into a 'mutant gene', and the produced outcome may or may not be in harmony with the other cells leading to diseases in our body. When there is a change in the coding, the body starts producing defective cells and to prevent the damage by these mutant cells, our defence system comes into play. Our immune system immediately tries to destroy those abnormal cells and the self-correction mechanism of our DNA, also tries to fix the faulty coding. When the assaulting stimulus persists for a longer period of time and our defence system fails, we become victim of that particular disease.

Our lifestyle and our immediate environment play a major role in altering our DNA codes and make us vulnerable to diseases. This is due to the information reaching the cell through its receptors, expresses the code for the disease written in the DNA. Cancer, diabetes, hypertension are few examples of our defective coding, which we express because of our self-mismanagement of the body.

For example, we have a strong belief that if a person is diabetic his children will become diabetic by default. As if, the child is a victim of his DNA. However, the new epigenetic research shows that, the person will not become diabetic until and unless he expresses his diabetic gene. The expression of genes depends on the signals from the environment. This is the reason; type II diabetic people, are mostly diagnosed for the first time when they are in an adverse physical and mental condition. Once the gene is expressed, disease sets in and the reverse is, also true. If we create a favourable environment for our cells, living a healthy life forever is practically possible. We can educate and empower people with these basic facts and convince them about the possibility of setting things back to normalcy by us. Once we understand this fact, the disease burden will decrease and living a healthy life will become a routine.

Quantum Health

Science has now proved it beyond doubt that the universe, is not made up of matter but of invisible vibrating energy. The things we see as solid are nothing but are immaterial force fields seen under an atomic microscope. However, physics is following the quantum principles since the time Einstein postulated the theory of relativity, but medicine is still in the Newtonian era. Albert

Einstein once told; "The field is the sole governing agency of the physical reality". What he meant for the 'field' is the invisible energy.

According the quantum theory, anything is possible and there can be many outcomes to any event or happenings. There are unlimited potential outcome to every situation. We are living in a quantum world, in which we all are inter connected and our energy are entangled. We cannot be separated from our immediate environment; in fact, we are an extension of our environment, which includes our thoughts, our belief systems, our lifestyle and the exposures to environmental pollutions. Out thought is the most potent vibration in this universe. The power of thoughts allows us to experience a higher richness of life and our higher self.

Dr. Bruce Lipton has rightly said, "The new biology moves us out of Victimhood into Mastery over our own health". We now have the power to alter our genetic expressions, by changing the way of thinking, good food habits and by improving our breathing quality. By educating people to empower themselves with the knowledge of epigenetic model of life, one day we will be able to change the course of diseases and live a longer and healthier life.

Experiencing the Vibration Journey

We are made up of trillions of cells. Cells are made of molecules. Molecules are made of atoms. Atoms are made of subatomic particles. These subatomic particles are nothing but vortices of energy that are constantly spinning and vibrating. Therefore, every atom has its own energy signature. We are nothing but unique energy bundles, radiating energy to our surroundings. Our energy waves are constantly interacting with the other source of energies and there is interference. This interference can be either constructive or destructive. This is the reason, we get the feelings of good or bad, whenever we are in contact with a person or a place, depending on the frequency they generate.

We can vibrate our atoms in a constructive way and magnify the amplitude of our vibrations at will and can remain healthy forever. This will help us to overcome illness, as the sick cells are vibrating in a lower frequency.

This is possible by the sounds described in our scriptures like Aum, Amen, Allah, Hmmm. Humming a mantra create vibration of a frequency of 432 Hz, which is the natural frequency of the universe. When we practice it, our cells also start vibrating with that frequency and bring health and happiness in our life.

Do It Now

Let us set a time of a day for Aum chanting. Early Morning is preferable. First, we have to choose a quiet place and have a comfortable position. Minimum 15 minutes is a good time to chant. Let us relax our whole body with the count of one, two, and three with breathing deep and our eyes closed.

Now let us chant Aum in a slow and rhythmic way when we exhale. "A" should pronounce like the letter 'a' in the word "saw", combined with the "U" sounding like letter 'u' in the word "put". Than blend "M" into the end like mmmm. The sound should be drawn from the naval and the vibration should rise upward until the nostril. Let us repeat it as long as we are comfortable.

CHAPTER IV

Care for Your Breath

For a purposeful life, we have to have a vision of a healthy body and mind,
with a mission to create a wonderful and happy world.

Author

I am a surgeon, and I have to deal with sick people. Every time I go for my ward round, the first thing I used to notice is, my patient's posture and the way they carry their body. During my postgraduate training, my professor and guide Dr. Saxena always insisted on getting the patients sit during the ward round and always asked us to stand behind the patients and pat on their back. By doing that simple procedure, the patient's respiration used to improve and the chest used to get free from secretions, which was mostly due to bad posture and inactivity. We could see the instant change of patient's expression after this simple procedure.

A proper breathing is regenerative and restorative. We breathe through a complex and highly sophisticated mechanical apparatus called respiratory system, controlled by the Autonomic nervous system through our respiratory centre present in brain. We are born to breathe fully. When we come to this world from mother's womb, we cry to take our first breath, which opens up the collapsed lungs for the first time. This first breath was natural, conscious and complete. We are born to breathe fully and effortlessly. We follow this natural pattern for a certain period of time, until the environment starts influencing our body and our mind. Over time, we accumulate stress and tension of our family and people surrounding us. We develop emotions like, love, anger, joy, hatred and feelings like pain and pleasure. These acquired behaviours gradually take away the expansiveness that we used to have, as a child. Then our breathing pattern becomes unconscious, small and shallow. We some time even stop to breathe, for a short period during stress and emotional outbursts. This is the cause of uneasiness, we feel during that period and our suffering starts by the discrepancy in the demand and supply of flow of blood, nutrients and vital energy to our brain.

We no more breathe consciously and restrict our breathing by tightening our muscles. This type of breathing affects our respiration, cardiovascular rhythm, our neuromuscular coordination, our gut functions and all other systems our body to a great extent. With a highly stressful environment, our biological rhythms of life gets restricted or distorted and leads us to an unhealthy and unconscious breathing pattern which allow us to survive but does not allow us to thrive.

This machine like any other mechanical apparatus needs lots of skill and knowledge to run it optimally. Unfortunately, the operative manual is never provided to us until we are ready to look for it and practice certain techniques. The most important factor is to direct our consciousness back to our breathing and learning to work with it. Lungs are one of the four motors of our body, which are directly controlled by our autonomic nervous system. The other three are our heart, Liver and kidney.

Breathing is automatic as Autonomic Nervous System (ANS) controls it. This is the only organ, on which we have a partial control.

Do we really know about this wonderful life-giving organ and use it to our advantage?

The secret of our energetic body is the amount of oxygen that gets in to our body for use in our cells. The more oxygen we breathe in to our lungs, the more energy we will have. The food molecules, which are absorbed into our bloodstream, do utilize the oxygen and releases energy when they are metabolized inside our cells. It is like a combustion engine and requires oxygen to produce energy.

We should know little about our lung anatomy. The organs of respiration consist of two lungs, one on either side of the chest and the air passages that lead to them. They are located in the upper thoracic cavity of the chest, one on each side of median line. The lungs tissue is pink in colour and is spongy, porous and their tissues are very elastic. The substance of the lungs contains innumerable air sacs, which contain air. The heart, great vessel, trachea, bronchi, food pipe, and lymphatic occupy the area between the lungs.

Anatomy

The air-passage consists of: (fig 1)

1. The nose
2. The pharynx or throat
3. The larynx or sounding box, which contains two vocal cords

4.   The trachea or windpipe

5.   The right and left bronchi and the smaller bronchial tubes

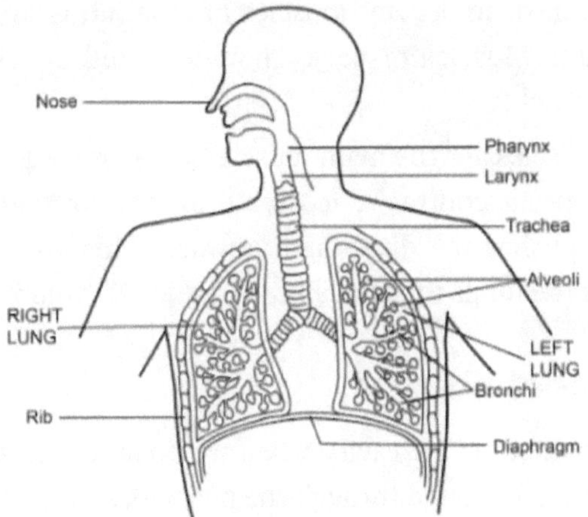

Figure 1

This part of the respiratory system does the work of a filter and as a humidifier. Air inside the passage does not take part in the gas exchange.

The air exchange apparatus consists of

1.   The Alveoli

2.   The capillaries

We have around 800 millions of alveoli or sacs of elastic tissue, which can expand like tiny balloons. Tiny capillaries, lined up on these alveolar wall and help in exchange of oxygen with poisonous metabolic by products like co2 and water. In a typical young adult male about 5 to 5.5 litres of air gets exchanged every Minute and in a female it is about 25 percent less.

The Muscles of Respiration Are

1.   Inter costal muscles

2.   Diaphragm

3.   Neck and shoulder muscles

4.   Abdominal muscles

Our lungs by itself are passive in nature. They inflate and deflate due to movements of walls of thoracic (chest) cavity causing pumping of air, to move in and out of lungs. The muscles of thorax are partly voluntary and partly involuntary. The most important muscles of respiration are the intercostals and the diaphragm. Muscles of neck, shoulders, and abdomen assist these muscles when needed.

Abdominal muscles are the main muscle for the forced exhalation. When the abdominal muscle contracts, it exerts inward pressure on abdominal viscera and thus pushes the diaphragm upward. This upward movement of diaphragm forces the lungs to expel air and reduce its volume.

Breathing Mechanisms

Air is drawn in to the thoracic cavity when we breathe. Air gushes in through the nose and after it has passed through the pharynx and larynx, it reaches into the trachea, then into the right and left bronchial tubes. The Bronchial tubes, are subdivide into innumerable smaller tubes called bronchioles, which are made up of fibrous muscular coat and ciliated mucous lining. The bronchioles terminate in minute subdivisions in the small air sacs of the lungs called alveoli, which the lungs contain millions. The air sacs of the lungs when spread out over an unbroken surface, would cover, an area of 1, 40,000 square feet.

Only 10% if the total respiratory capacity is used during each breath, in a quiet respiration. *The catch point is; this breathing volume can be increased by practice, so that our cells can get more oxygen and remain healthy for a longer period.* Another paradox about the gaseous exchange is that, the distribution of blood in the lung is gravity dependent. Therefore, the base of the lungs near the diaphragm gets more flow then the apex. On the other hand, alveolar flow of air is more in the upper portion of lung, due to its natural property. By changing the breathing pattern, we can direct the flow of oxygen to the lower portion of the lungs.

Nose the Filter

The Nostrils are the control mechanism for the flow of breath and has direct connection to the brain. These are the doorway to the mind body system. It is more than just a pathway to air. They are lined by coarse hairs, which act as a filter against dusts and other foreign bodies. The mucous lining of the nostrils helps to clean, humidify and regulates the temperature of the air entering the lung. There are approximately 5 million nerve receptors within the olfactory bulb, which conduct impulses to the portion of the brain lying directly over the nasal cavity. During inhalation, the flow of air in each nostril stimulates specific unilateral autonomic nerve centres lying within and beneath the mucous membranes, which influences the autonomic process of respiration, digestion, circulation etc. The nose apart from its function as an air conditioner, heater, filter, and moisturizer, it has direct effect on physical, mental, emotional, psychic, and spiritual state.

Inhalation

Inhalation is produced by contraction of the diaphragm. When contracted the diaphragm flattens out and moves downward, resulting in an increase in the volume of thoracic cavity. This generates a negative pressure and draws air into the lungs. With a complete and healthy breath, the diaphragm easily expands downward along with the lower lobes of lungs. For this to happen, our body should be in a relaxed state of mind, as stress causes our muscles to be tight and immovable for a certain period. Inhalation brings in oxygen and it is energizing and extroverting. This stimulates sympathetic nervous system and promotes catabolism. Our diaphragmatic action provides an important massage to both chest and abdominal organs like heart, stomach, intestines, liver, spleen, pancreatic and kidney. This action stimulates blood circulation and helps our digestion, assimilation and excretion process, which are essential for maintaining life and health.

Exhalation

When we breathe out, or exhale, our diaphragm relaxes and moves upward into the chest cavity. The intercostals muscles between the ribs also relax to reduce the space in the chest cavity.

As the space in the chest cavity gets smaller, the carbon dioxide and water vapour are forced out of the lungs, through our windpipe. This is purifying and introverting. This stimulates parasympathetic nervous system and promotes anabolism.

Physiology

Lung purifies the blood. The impure blood, (blue in colour) mixed with the waste matter of the system reaches the heart through the venous route. The heart then sends it to the lung through the right ventricle, where it is allowed to mix, with the oxygen we have inhaled from the atmosphere. In these millions of tiny alveoli of the lungs, the purification of the impure blood takes place through the hair like blood vessels called pulmonary capillaries. During this contact period, the impure blood takes up oxygen and begins its arterial journey, and becomes bright red. The purified blood reaches left ventricle through four pulmonary veins and left auricle. Left ventricle then distributes the purified, life enriched blood throughout the body by its pumping mechanism, through the biggest artery Aorta. It is estimated that in a day 35000 pints of blood traverse the capillaries of lungs for purification.

What Affects Our Respiration?

As our breathing is controlled by autonomic nervous system, the quality of it changes with the sympathetic and parasympathetic activities occurring in our bodies. With the activation of sympathetic nervous system, our body goes to a protective mode where we breathe faster to fulfil the oxygen demand of the body. During parasympathetic activity body goes to growth mode and our respiration becomes slow and deep.

How Breathing Affect the Rest of the System?

Our breathing is partially controlled by involuntary and partially by voluntary nervous system. In normal circumstances, nervous control is unconscious or involuntary. A quiet breathing is sufficient to maintain arterial oxygen and carbon dioxide level. However when there is a change in the body's biomechanical rhythm due to wide range of physiological, environmental and pathological conditions, the rate and depth of respiration changes to bring back the homeostasis of the body. Our emotions like anger, happiness, excitement, depressions and sensory impulses like pain, physical exercises affect our breathing pattern. Also some other factors like, climatic changes, state of mind, medications, environmental temperatures etc alters our breathing process.

What Breathing Does?

The oxygen present in the atmosphere is the most important molecule for the maintenance of life. Our respiration is all about bringing oxygen from atmosphere into the lungs, which purifies the blood and supplies it to our cells for utilization. Our respiration also eliminates the toxic by-products like carbon dioxide and water out of the body. This exchange occurs at the alveoli during the period of pause between inhalation and exhalation. Therefore, this phase of contact is the most vital part of the respiration. As the respiration is partially voluntary, we can improve our exchange period by following certain technical rules.

Most of us are not aware that we breathe very poorly. In this fast moving world of distractions, poor breathing is the biggest disease creator. Lack of knowledge about proper ways of breathing, leads us to become habitual chest breather or indulge us in breathing, very fast and shallow. If we look around, we will find people everywhere with stiff and tight body, running after their ambitions. Our ancient scriptures and many scientific studies done throughout the world, has already proved that this type of effortless or unconscious breathing habits can lead us to allure most of the chronic health problems. Poor or shallow breathing means less contact time for diffusion of gases at the alveolar levels. This is directly responsible for poor oxygen supply to thencells, which ultimately in due course of time become unhealthy and diseases sets in.

By controlling our breathing pattern, we shift ourselves from operating in a stress mode to a mode of relaxation and alertness. This altered relaxed mode promotes the synthesis of molecules, responsible for our growth and repair and increase the production of our protector immune cells. This state enhances our cellular, hormonal and psychological well-being. Mind becomes clearer and emotions become more balanced through calm and regular breathing. This is conducive to health, well-being, and sense of inner peace. Breathing is one of the many unconscious processes of the body that can be voluntarily controlled.

What Is Good Breathing?

When we breathe consciously and completely and utilize the full capacity of the lungs, it is considered a good breathing. A correct breathing improves one's physical and mental well-being. All of our ancient practices like yoga, qigong, etc gave maximum importance to conscious breathing. Practicing the methods mentioned above develop good breathing habits.

Conscious Breathing

The first step of conscious breathing is to become more aware of the breathing process. Though this sounds simple, it needs a lots of practice. Counting the breath and concentrating on the inhalation and exhalation create awareness about our own breathing. We can practice it by sitting comfortably or in a laid down position. Without disturbing our natural rhythms, we just have to be aware of every breath. Just observe the flow, whether it is slow or fast, shallow or deep, regular or irregular. This awareness on breathing brings relaxation and eases tension. We can deepen our awareness on the nostrils, on windpipe, on the passing of air to our lungs and again the exhalation of air through the same root. We can be aware of the movement of our diaphragm moving downwards as we inhale and upward as we exhale.

Types of Breathing

1. Abdominal

2. Thoracic or chest

3. Clavicular or shoulder

Abdominal Breathing

Abdominal breathing is due to the downward movement of diaphragmatic muscle during inhalation and upward on exhalation. This type of breathing is an integral part of deep breathing. It should be incorporated in our daily life, so that it becomes a habit. Poor posture, stress, tight clothing, sudden emotional outbursts etc. prevents abdominal breathing. A mastery over this technique can bring a wonderful physical and mental well-being. Abdominal breathing has a parasympathetic cardiovascular component, which helps us calm down and reduces our stress level.

This type of breathing increases the lung capacity and helps in absorbing more oxygen, so that it can fulfil the extra demand created by the body in certain activities like sports and exercise.

In abdominal breathing diaphragm is in motion, it massages the abdominal organs and abdominal muscles. This movement increases the blood circulation of the organs and improves the digestive, metabolic and excretory functions. *Deep breathing releases chemicals like endorphins into our circulation.* Endorphin is a wonderful neuropeptide, known as natural painkiller and reduces anxiety and fear.

Deep breathing reduces the dead space of the respiratory apparatus and increases the efficiency of gas exchange through the increased flow of blood in the lower lobes of the lungs. Deep breathing also assists in the return flow of blood from the lower part of body to the heart.

Chest Breathing

This is also known as thoracic breathing and produced by expansion and contraction of rib cage. It is a less efficient type of breathing but required during increased physical activity. There is a horizontal expansion of the lung and some of the alveoli remain closed and collect secretions, causing them to become prone to diseases. This is the most common type of breathing when we are in stress to compensate the oxygen requirement of the body. About 20% or more of population are habitual chest breather. Chest breathing has an increased sympathetic dominance, which leads to increase in heart rate and cardiac output. This also decreases the blood flow to heart and brain and is the cause of major cardiac problems.

Clavicular Breathing

This type of breathing takes little effort and ventilates the upper lobes. This type of breathing is found as a component of yogic breathing, at the final stage of total rib expansion. Mostly occurs during sobbing or asthma attack.

Yogic Breathing

Yogic breathing or Pranayama is the recommendation of the **"Care for your health"**.

A yogic breathing is a combination of all these three types of breathing mentioned above. It increases the ventilation by increasing the volume of air in both the expanded lungs and increases the exchange time for the gas. In yogic breathing, the lungs are stretched to maximum capacity in both inhalation and exhalation. In this type, the inhalation begin from the Lower lobe and completes at the upper lobe. In exhalation, the process is just reverse. Practicing yogic breathing can correct the poor breathing habits and increase the oxygen intake. This is a conscious breathing, controlled by our will. Conscious breathing is registered in the frontal brain.

Deep breathing practice is a basic component for **caring of your health,** as 'breathing is life'. Unfortunately, most of us breathe unconsciously because we lack the proper knowledge. Few of us who perform the breathing practices, do it incorrectly, as we are not aware of the basic breathing mechanism and its benefits. Through this chapter, I have given brief descriptions and this will ignite your mind to learn more by further study of literature. Yoga, Qi gong, meditation are based on slow breathing.

Pranayama is the science of breathing developed by great yogis to attain balance in the body and control the mind. It has three components, *Inhalation, retention and exhalation.* According to **Maharshi Patanjali,** *'pranayama is the pause in the movement of inhalation and exhalation'.* In reality, pranayama is only **retention** as it allows a longer period for exchange of oxygen and carbon dioxide in the cells. All of our organs function optimally because there cells get the energy from the food we eat and the oxygen we inhale. So indirectly, a yogic breathing helps to keep our cells healthy and vibrant.

The exercises of pranayama include all the three types of breathing (deep, rapid and slow). The chest is opened to its fullest and lung is stretched to its maximum. With regular practice, it strengthens the muscles of breathing and increases the elasticity of lung tissues. The practice of pranayama allows more time for oxygen to mix with the blood and exchange with the metabolic by products, leading to elimination through breathing and other organs.

All the abdominal organs like liver, kidney, spleen, pancreas etc. gets more blood supply because of the massage, generated by the increased movement of diaphragm and abdominal muscle. This makes the digestive system more efficient and prepares it for better absorption of nutrients.

Numerous studies on deep breathing, shows that slow, deep and long breathe gives rest to the heart. Breathing in a ratio of 1:2 relaxes the coronary muscle without reducing the oxygen supply to brain or body tissue. Deep breathing during pranayama gently massages the coronary muscle and improves the coronary circulation. Pranayama gives proper training to the coronary circulation of the person.

Pranayama influences our endocrine system significantly. During pranayama, the blood supply to the organs become very rapid and quality of the blood is also very rich in oxygen. This enhances the functionality of the gland and helps to balance the system.

The neuronal activities of the brain become more rhythmical and regulated when we breathe slowly and deeply, as in Pranayama. Our activities and behaviours are nothing but the memories stored in our brain. Practicing Pranayama brings a great balance between both hemispheres.

Breathing Principles

I have seen the difference in the healing process among my patients depending on their type of respiration. Most of us are not good at using our respiratory system to its maximum. Breathing is our life, and doing this properly is the secret to a healthy body. Breathing is a natural process and the normal rate is about 15 breaths per minute, 900 breaths per hour and 21600 breaths per day. The breath rate is inversely proportional to the longevity of a person, more respiratory rates lead to a decreased life span. Swami Sivananda once said, "A yogi measures the span of life by the numbers of breath not by the numbers of years".

Few tips to people interested to do deep breathing exercises

1. Never do it without fully knowing the basic physiology behind it.

2. To reap the benefit we have to do it regularly and Fix a time for it.

3. Breath control means duration, depth, and force of inhalation, retentins and exhalations.

4. Body awareness is necessary before starting pranayama. The air should be inhaled slowly with awareness. The air should be retained properly with awareness. The air should be exhaled slowly with awareness.

5. We should always do it with proper ratio of inhalation, retention and exhalation.

6. We should not do any breathing practice randomly, by watching videos or prompted by some well-wisher. Learn from a qualified teacher.

7. Mindfulness breathing is doing deep breathing while we are doing our normal household works. We should do inhalation and exhalation attentively with the movement of abdomen.

8. We should keep the spine and head in one line.

My Experience with Breathing

Human physiology was the subject we were taught in our first year of the medical curriculum. By the time we were prepared to serve as trained physicians, we were very much acquainted with the physiological changes of the diseases rather than health. During initial period of my practice, I was not giving time for myself due to heavy workload. One day, while climbing the staircase I felt tired and had shortness of breath. That was the time, I felt something was wrong, in the way I was living my life. I started doing my deep breathing exercise 10 years back and today I can climb the stair without any problem. This is the power of breathing. I always teach my patients the basic breathing technique before and after operation. This technique ia a wonderful wound healer.

Chapter V

Care for Your Heart

We all are born healthy, but the bitter truth is that, none of us will remain healthy, until and unless we sincerely work towards a healthy lifestyle by adopting good habits and following certain rules.

Author

"Heart", the moment this word comes to our mind, feelings of love, compassion, joy, and fulfilment comes to our mind, with an added fear of dysfunctioning of the heart causing death. It is the emotional organ of our body, although emotions do not originate from the heart. Heart plays an important role in the overall maintenance of our health. It is the first functional organ in human embryo, formed by 4 weeks of development. Right from the moment, our heart is formed up until we die, it constantly serves us without taking rest for a single moment. If a person lives for about 75 years and with a heart rate of 75/min, his heart will beat for approximately 3,000,000,000 times. It is linked to the whole of the body in such a way that, it is affected by any change or dysfunction of other part of the body and vice versa. It is the organ, which is formed before our brain development starts, so it is the most primitive organ. The intelligence of our heart is superior to other organs.

In our modern day living, we are constantly updated with information about the heart diseases, its complications and the database of the epidemiology. Though we call it information and awareness, this type of activities make the society more disease conscious and sick. Very few of the information we gather is about keeping our heart strong and to remain healthy throughout the life. Heart is the place where the body, the mind and the spirit all converge. This book is an attempt to make you more health conscious and help you to maintain a healthy heart.

As a consultant, I used to get many such queries from my patients regarding their heart conditions, but had to refuse patients with those cardiac diseases for surgery, due to my centre's limitations. These queries of my patients led me to understand the intricacies, related to the heart and analyze it more closely. And the conclusion of my findings verified that, it is possible

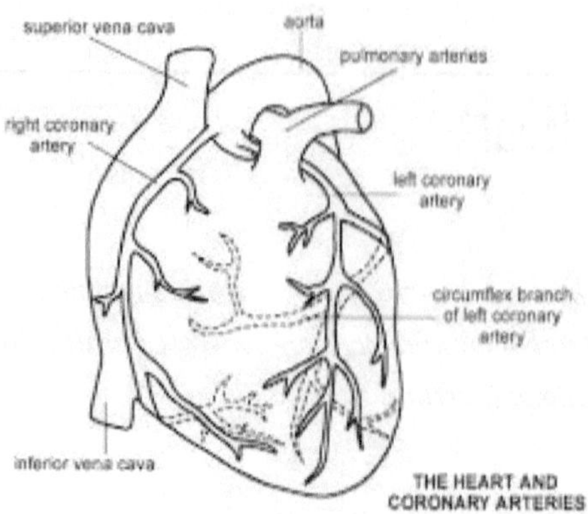

Figure 2

to remain healthy forever with a young heart till we die. My journey into this area of preventive aspect of medicine started in a very unusual way. 15 years of my practice as a solo consultant in a private hospital in India had made my life a mess. Doing 6 to 10 surgeries a day, outpatient examinations, follow up of old cases, ward dressings, ward rounds used to consume about 13 to 15 hrs a day. The aggressiveness and dedication towards my work gave me a special status in the society but it gradually made me sick from inside. This realization came to me in the year 2010 when I got an ECG done, because I felt little uncomfortable at the left side of my chest. It turned out to be abnormal and as usual, I was put into many more investigations.

This was the first time I did introspected on my life style and started acknowledging the abuse I did to my body. No exercises, missed lunch, less sleep, high stress are few of the factors I could pinpoint as the cause of my problem. After all the tests, I was given a clean chit that I did not have any major problem. My realization forced me to change my lifestyle and I started my journey into wellness. It has worked for me and I assure, it would work on anybody who will follow the right path leading to a healthy heart, like I did.

We are born healthy. We have an organ, which serves us till our death. It has an inherent capacity to remain healthy and adopt tackling adverse situations to a certain extent. It also gives enough warnings to keep us updated, about its condition every now and then. When we fail to perceive the warning signs and adopt a careless attitude, it starts failing and we land up in an unwarranted and unpleasant critical condition.

Remaining healthy is our responsibility. We should be aware of the power we have and the basic knowledge about our heart and the factors responsible for the deterioration of our heart health. This will empower us to take preventive steps to stop the ongoing damage. This chapter will elaborate on this aspect of heart care.

Anatomy and Function

Our heart is the most unselfish organ of our body as it not only does good by supplying oxygen rich pure blood to every cells of our body, but also carries back the toxic by-product for removal, through our excretory organs like lungs, kidneys and skin. When our body gets disturbed, it is the heart, which tries to balance it by increasing or decreasing heart rate. It also supplies blood to its own cells through two main tubes called left and right coronary arteries. Due to our inappropriate behaviour and abuse to our system, the innocent heart bears the burden and starts suffering. With the suffering of our heart, we suffer and the ultimate result is death.

Pathology

Our heart suffers from mainly two type of pathology.

One is the blockage of the coronary vessels because of narrowing. This narrowing prevents the heart from getting its blood supply and starts crying for the nutrients. Many of the times, it starts developing small tributaries, which supply blood to the deprived part to some extent and survive. When there is complete absence of blood supplies to a big portion of the heart, it stops functioning and death occurs. The most interesting part of this is that we are responsible for this type of narrowing of lumen of blood vessels and we have the power to dismantle the block and regain life. This will happen when we start taking care of our health.

The second cause is the disturbance in the electrical circuit of the heart, due to which the heart beats in irregular manner. This leads to arrhythmias, and unwanted heartbeats, causing abnormal heart functioning and failure. The causes of this type of irregularities are mostly the way we live our life, our stress level and our emotions. This can be taken care by changing our lifestyle.

Another variety of heart pathology is the rise of blood pressure where the force of blood against the artery walls is too high. This rise of blood pressure is due to the resistance our blood vessels give to the flow of blood when our heart pumps blood through narrowed or less elastic vessels. This pathology of heart may be **primary** and develop gradually over a period of time, known as *essential hypertension.* The **secondary** variety is due to some existing pathology like sleep apnoea, kidney problems, adrenal gland tumour, thyroid problems, certain medicines, smoking and other drug abuse. Incidence of all of these can be minimized with certain way of changing our lifestyle.

Apart from theses three variety, the other pathological variety is cardiomyopathy, where the heart muscle becomes diseased and ultimately it fails to serve properly. When the heart muscles become thicker,it is known as hypertrophic cardiomyopathy. When the chamber becomes bigger, it is known as dilated cardiomyopathy. In some variety of cardiomyopathy the heart chamber stiffens, and is known as restrictive cardiomyopathy. These are nothing but the abnormal cardiac cell dysfunction, resulting from our careless lifestyle.

Factors Responsible for Heart Disorder

Most of the heart pathologies as described above are due to few factors as described below.

A. Cholesterol Story

"Care for your heart" is all about the knowledge of cholesterol, as it is the most common cause of CAD (Coronary Artery Diseases). Cholesterol is a waxy material found in our food rich in fats. Milk and milk products, eggs, meat, fish etc are rich in cholesterol. It is required for formation of many essential molecules in our body like, vitamin D, bile acids, sex hormones, nerve sheath and cell membranes etc. A large proportion of cholesterol is formed in our liver and released into intestine. Ninety percent of these again gets absorbed through intestines and reach the bloodstream. As cholesterol is not water soluble, it forms a water-soluble compound called chylomicron, by combining with protein and fat molecules. These chylomicrons or lipoproteins carry cholesterol through bloodstream to different parts of the body. The different types of lipoproteins are:

1. VLDL – (very low-density lipoprotein): It contains the highest amount of triglycerides as it carries into our bloodstream.

2. LDL – It is (low-density lipoprotein) also known as BAD CHOLESTEROL. It is a product of VLDL, after the removal of triglycerides and mostly derived from Trans fats and saturated fats. Excessive accumulation of LDL in blood results in clogging and narrowing of the blood vessels. LDL level

should not exceed 130 mg. It has been proved that stress increases the LDL level and stress reduction decreases the level.

3. HDL – It is (High-density lipoprotein) also known as GOOD CHOLESTEROL. During its formation, it collects cholesterols from the blood, and transports them to liver, from where the cholesterol is secreted in the bile. Therefore, it plays the role of a cholesterol cleanser in the body. The normal level of the HDL in male is between 36–45 mg and female 40–60 mg. The more the HDL, the lesser the ratio and safer we are. Exercise increases the HDL level and smoking decreases the level.

4. TRIGLYCERIDES – These are the types of fat produced by the liver. Triglycerides are the main constituents of body fat in human beings. When we eat, our body converts extra calories, which does not have any use, converts into Triglycerides. When we need energy, our body converts them in to energy for use in-between meals. This has maximum contribution for the hardening of arterial wall.

Taking care of your heart is taking care of your cholesterol. The basic knowledge about the normal values is important, as we have to adjust our food habits to maintain our cholesterol level within these parameters.

Desired Cholesterol Level

serum lipids	normal	Low risk	Borderline	High risk
VLDL	10–30 mg/dl	<30 mg/dl		
LDL	80–150 mg/dl	<130 mg/dl	130–160	>160
HDL	150–200 mg/dl	>60	35–60	<35
TOTAL CHOLESTEROL	150–200 mg/dl	<200	200–240	>240
SERUM TRIGLYCERIDES	50–150 mg/dl	<200	200–499	>500

Note:

Ratio of total cholesterol to HDL: - The most important is the **ratio** of total cholesterol to HDL. A ratio of 4.5 and lower is considered normal and associated with low cardiac risk. For example, if my total cholesterol is 180 and my HDL is 40, my ratio will be

$$\frac{\text{Total cholesterol (180)}}{\text{HDL cholesterol (40)}} = 4.5$$

This has borderline risk case, although both the parameters are within normal limits.

The Story

High cholesterol level in our blood is primarily responsible for coronary artery diseases in human being where there is gradual clogging and blockage of coronary arteries. We call it atherosclerosis and are due to deposition of fat and cholesterol in the wall of arteries. Of all cholesterol, LDL known as bad cholesterol is the most dangerous one, as it is responsible for maximum deposits of plaques in the arterial lumen. Patients get heart attacks when clots block the narrowed coronary arteries. Clot formation occurs when the blood is exposed to a ruptured plaque within the arterial wall. This is nothing but the local reaction to bleeding.

Many genetic factors and environmental risk factors can increase or decrease the blood cholesterol levels. In 1985, Nobel Prize winner Dr. Michel Brown and Joseph Goldstein discovered LDL cholesterol receptors. It was then identified that the more cholesterol receptors we have, the more efficiently we can metabolize and remove cholesterol from our blood. The fewer cholesterol receptors we have, the more our cholesterol level will rise with fewer intakes of fatty diets.

Causes of High Cholesterol

1. Hereditary

Some genetic lipoprotein disorders, like familial hyperlipidemia, familial hypertriglyceridemia, and familial hypercholesterolemiaare genetically linked, and consist of 1-5% of the total population. Unfortunately, we do not have much option to reduce this type of problem except a very sincere lifestyle.

2. Stress

Stress puts our body into the fight or flight mode. When we enter into this mode, our body responds to it by secreting increased volume of pituitary, adrenal and thyroid hormones. Our body requires these chemicals whenever we are in danger. These chemicals are required for muscle contraction and increasing heart rate. When we are in stress for a longer period, these same hormones are being used for increased fat deposits and high triglycerides formation

3. Addiction

Addiction to tea and coffee, tobacco, alcohol, soft drinks are the new age cause of increased cholesterol. Caffeine present in tea, coffee and cold drinks is the main culprit in raising the cholesterol level in our body. Many studies, throughout the world have proved that increased consumption of tea and coffee increases the risk of heart diseases. Excessive caffeine can cause irregular heartbeats leading to cardiac arrhythmia. Limiting the intake of tea and coffee is the recommendation for the "Care for your heart" instruction. Smoking has been linked to heart diseases since long. It increases the bad cholesterol LDL level.

4. Obesity

Obese persons have high blood cholesterol. Triglycerides and LDL levels are very high and HDL cholesterol level is low. It is the bad food habit of consuming excessive amount of calories, saturated fats and cholesterol, which are responsible for high blood fat level. Many studies have proved that, choosing active lifestyle, regular exercise and weight reduction can reduce the blood cholesterol and prevent cardiac deaths.

5. Diseases Responsible for High Cholesterol

Diabetes, high blood pressure, thyroid disorders, kidney diseases and pancreatic diseases are associated with high cholesterol level. High Blood pressure injures the coronary artery lining by the direct hitting of blood on the side of its wall with increased force. Inflammatory reactions set in due to the injury and plaque formation starts resulting in narrowing of lumen. This starts a cyclical phenomenon. The blood pressure further increases to overcome the resistance provided by the narrowed vessels. Most of the diseases need a meticulous care. To keep the rise of cholesterol in all these disease conditions under control, we need adequate awareness and care.

6. Drugs

Certain drugs can cause the cholesterol level to rise to an alarming level. The drugs used to increase your urine output, known as diuretic, Beta blockers, the most common medicines used to control blood pressure and anabolic steroids increase our total cholesterol and LDL and triglyceride level. We have to be careful in taking these medications and adopt a lifestyle, which will prevent these diseases to escalate.

7. Physical Inactivity

Physical inactivity is a new world problem and is comparable with smoking. With the development of modern technology and the increase in the availability of things near our home, our lifestyle becomes more sedentary. This inactivity then leads to obesity, high cholesterol and increase in blood pressure.

B. Blood Pressure Story

High Blood pressure injures the coronary artery lining by the direct hitting of the blood on the side of its wall with increase force. An inflammatory reaction sets in due to the injury and plaque formation starts resulting in narrowing of lumen. This starts a cyclical phenomenon. The blood pressure further increases to overcome the resistance provided by the narrowed vessels

C. Contraction Story

Heart muscles can get damaged independent of coronary blood flow. Here due to constant stressful circumstances, the heart muscle fibres fails to relax and constrict to the point, that it damages itself. Our stress hormones adrenaline and steroids causes the coronary arteries to constrict and there is a cry for oxygen. This leads to weakening of heart muscles and dilatation of heart. This condition is known as cardiomyopathy in which the heart's pumping capability decreases and heart failure sets in.

D. Nicotine Story

The nicotine present in the tobacco causes direct damage to the lining of blood vessels and induces inflammation, which in turn leads to clogging of arteries and clot formation. Nicotine damages the platelets of our blood and these damaged platelets aggravates the clot formation in heart vessels. Smoking increases the level of our stress chemical levels, which causes our heart to beat faster and increases its oxygen consumption. When the stressful environment persists for a longer period, these chemicals irritate the heart muscles and force the heart to beat irregularly. Carbon monoxide present in the smoke competes with the oxygen, for haemoglobin and is carried to all over the body. So when the carbon monoxide percentage increases the supplied areas becomes deprived of oxygen and start functioning abnormally.

E. Diet Story

Food rich in saturated fats and cholesterol are the building blocks for coronary atherosclerosis. The most important fact is that diet affects the heart very quickly. A diet rich in high cholesterol can immediately release the hormone thromboxane and can cause the artery to constrict and blood to clot faster. This is the reason people get chest pain immediately after eating foods rich in fat in a party. The reverse is also true. If we change our diet to low fat and other lifestyle changes, the reversal of heart disease can occur within few months.

F. Story of Salt and Sugar

Salt is not that bad, as it is perceived to be, a culprit, in individual with hypertension. Less than one fourth of people, who are hypertensive, are salt responsive. Our body retains water in response to the salt present, to maintain a homeostasis. Therefore, it increases the water volume of our body and the excess salt and water is again excreted out through Kidney and sweat glands. Restriction of salt is advisable to persons having problems where there is less excretion of water, like in congestive heart failure and kidney diseases.

When a healthy individual eat refined sugar, there is a sudden rise of sugar level and pancreas respond quickly by secreting insulin, which helps to utilize the glucose by cells. Sugar is linked to heart disease poorly except the time we consume refined sugar with food rich with fat.

Care for Your Heart Is the Care for Your Cholesterols

Most of the factors responsible for heart disease are preventable and many of the heart conditions are reversible. Dr. Dean Ornish MD, a well known cardiologist of San Francisco, author of the best seller "Program for Reversing Heart disease " has documented that, Coronary Artery Diseases can be corrected and blocks can be cleared by adopting certain habits. According to him taking care of your heart is all about how to enjoy living rather than how to avoid dying, how to relax rather than not how to be lethargic and how to manage stress, not how to avoid it, how to live in this world more fully, rather than how to withdraw from it. He describes the technological interventions in cardiovascular diseases, as a half -hearted approach. It has its own limitations and bypasses the underlying causes of the problem.

He stated differently and instead of bypassing the problem, he emphasized on the change in lifestyle, which seemed to be the cause of their heart disease. The results were encouraging, and the results were more than expected. Initially they were expecting good results in younger age groups and with less advance disease, but to their surprise the most severely blocked arteries are the one that showed the maximum reversal.

Dr. Ornish has clearly emphasized on the fact that, though cholesterol is very important, it is not the whole story. High blood pressure, smoking, lack of exercise are the other factors associated with heart diseases amount to only 50%of the heart disease we see. During his studies, he was convinced that the factors like, emotional stress, perceived isolation, lack of social support, low self-esteem amounts to other half of the disease contributors.

Ways to Have a Healthy Heart

"Care for your heart" recommendations;

1. Food Habits

The food we eat play a major role in maintaining our heart health. The type of food you eat is more important than the amount of food you eat. Low fat vegetarian diet has shown remarkable results in reversing the heart blockage in all age groups in different studies. If we want to keep ourselves healthy throughout our life then we have to adopt a food habit of low fat and cholesterol and stick to it by the time we are in our late thirties. The oil to be used must be unsaturated fat. Dietary modifications also help in reducing the risk of other degenerative diseases including high blood pressure, diabetes, osteoporosis, and cancer. *'Care for your heart' does not advocate dieting or deprivation of food anymore.* Recommendation is to eat variety of food, so that the basic requirements of vitamins and amino acids reach our body.

Dr. Dean Ornish in his reversal diet recommends

- Ten percent fat, in the form of unsaturated oil as cooking medium and skimmed milk. Remember, fat by itself is not bad but too much of fat is the problem. Approximately 14 grams of fat per day fulfil the requirements of our body. 1 tablespoon is equivalent to 14 grams of fat.

All oils contain all the three variety of fats. If we take more of olive oil, which contains very less saturated fat, it will raise our cholesterol level significantly. It is because more oil will raise the percentage of saturated fat of olive oil.

- We should take 70 to 75 percent complex carbohydrates in the form of grains, beans, vegetables, fruits.

- 10 to 20% proteins Rice (grains) and beans (legume) provides a complete protein menu for an individual. The ideal proportion is two third grains and one third legume. Egg white is an example of complete proteins.

- He advocates less than 5 mg of cholesterol per day.

2. Exercise

Care For your heart recommends regular exercise as a mandatory activity in daily routines. Today's sedentary lifestyle is the primary cause for the rise of heart problems throughout the world. Technology has brought comfort to our life and with it has made us lazy. Every one of us knows regular exercise is good for us but only a small number of them do it. Half of the people do it for the sake of doing it, without the proper knowledge about the way it should be done. In my practice as a consultant, I see a good number of people, who are sick because they do it improperly. *Exercise for your heart should be a ritual, to be done every day with an intention to spend rest of our life healthy with a properly functioning heart.*

Exercising for a healthy heart is the talk of the time. *Exercise can train and strengthen our heart muscle, like any other type of muscle.*The only difference is that it cannot be trained directly as the heart muscles are involuntary. It can be trained indirectly by working on our peripheral muscle mass. The aim of exercise for heart health is to reduce cardiovascular risk among general mass, reduce disability and promote an active lifestyle for people suffering from cardiac diseases. Regular exercise improves our cardiac muscle, which then pumps out the blood more efficiently. *For the improvement of heart health, we need both aerobics and strength training.*

No exercise should be done when we are tired or when we are drained of our energy. Moderate exercise strengthens the immune system and energizes our body, where as excessive exercise depress the immune function. We should take low Glycemic Index food like banana or an apple before going for aerobic exercise. Drinking water as per our need is very important. Whenever we are going for an early morning walk or schedule our training session in the morning, we should prepare with low GI food like bananas, 25 minutes to 30 minutes before exercise.

Any exercise program should precede, by a good warm up period. Warming up increases the blood flow to the muscles, loosen up surrounding connective tissues. This prevents injury and reduces the risk of getting pull and tear of muscles, tendons and ligaments. Warm up exercises includes stretching of body parts and joints.

The key to aerobic or cardio exercise is to be within the target heart rate for getting maximum benefit out of it. Brisk Walking, jogging, cycling, swimming are some of the aerobics exercise we can do regularly.

Calculating Heart Rate

Maximum heart rate (MHR) = 220 – Age [Beats per minute]

Target heart rate (THR) = 60% to 70% of MHR.

In the beginning, our target heart rate should not be more than 60% of the MHR. We should calculate the pulse rate by palpating the pulsation of our radial artery. Gradually we should reach 70% to 75% of the MHR. Athletes can go up to 80% of MRH.

Care for health advocate walking as the best aerobic exercise we can do as it can be done by anyone. It is practical, cheap, and effective. Unfit person should do workout 50 percent to 60 percent of the maximum heart rate. Knowing the pulse rate during exercise helps us to stay in the target zone. In this zone, our heart and lungs work optimally to meet the body's demand for oxygen. Aerobic exercise is to be performed minimum of 25 to 30 minutes a day and 5 days a week. If done sincerely, it will strengthen the heart muscle and increase the lung capacity.

FITT Formula for Exercising

It is a way to monitor our exercise program.

F. Frequency

How many days in a week should we exercise? For a better response from the exercise we do, the frequency of the exercise sessions has to be planned properly and followed up regularly. Recommendation is 5 to 6 time per week. Depending on our current fitness level and our engagements, we have to plan so that we can follow it regularly

I. Intensity

Refers to high intensity or low intensity exercise we are planning to do to reach our exercise goal. Intensity of an exercise is monitored mostly through heart rate. It can be measured through Rated perceived exertion (RPE)

T. Time

This is to decide how much time we are doing and at what intervals. Recommendation time is 60 minutes maximum. For cardiovascular fitness 30 minutes of exercise is enough. For strength building, this gets replaced by sets and repetitions.

T. Type

Refers to choices of what type of exercise activity we are doing to meet our exercise goal. We have to choose among, walking, jogging, swimming, cycling, or resistance training.

Brain Derived Neurotrophic Factor (BDNF)

When we exercise, the body as a whole goes in to an energy generating mode. From our toes to the brain cells, all gets an increased supply of power and activate themselves for a quick start. Somebody has rightly said, "When we exercise, we are not only exercising our muscles, we are also training our DNA to work better and in a more efficient manner". Studies showed that the powerhouse of our cells, 'The mitochondria' grow in size and become more active during exercise. We are like rechargeable batteries, the more we are active, the more our mitochondria get recharged, and the more we are energized. This also activates the proteins responsible for making the brain active, by a mechanism called synaptic plasticity. This is due to a molecule called Brain Derived Neurotrophic Factor (BNDF). Exercise boosts BNDF production, and the level remains elevated for a full day after a moderate exercise session.

Exercise makes our lungs more efficient in oxygen exchange through diffusion, as heart pumps more blood to meet the demand. Our cells are now flooded with more raw materials for energy production. As the body temperature increases due to release of energy, there will be dilatation of peripheral vessels resulting in lowering of blood pressure. With time, there will be development of new capillaries network for better tissue perfusion. Exercises also renew the mitochondrial structures by reducing the damage caused by free radicals generation.

Walking

Walking is the most common exercise people do, as it is natural, inexpensive and suit to all groups of people. Every day I meet people who are the regular Walker, with lots of queries and dissatisfactions. The most common complain they have is a very unique one. "Why after doing regular exercise, I am not getting my health benefit and becoming sick frequently? Whenever I get such queries, I Just ask them to describe the way they perform the walking. Most of the time, I get an answer, which used to be just opposite to the way we should be walking for a healthy life. We should know the basics of walking, to reap the maximum benefit from walking exercise.

The first step is to set a clear goal for our walking exercise. We have to find out the reason for choosing walking as an exercise for us. Most commonly, we chose for remaining *healthy and physically active*. The term physical activity is synonyms with movement, in which the goal is to sustain daily living and recreation. The example is moving around to complete our daily routine works, may be at office or at home.

For a person having fitness as a goal, simple walking alone is not sufficient. To keep ourselves *healthy and fit* means keeping trillions of our cells healthy by making sure that every cell gets the nutrients and the oxygen properly for its functioning. This is possible when our walking goal meets all the criteria of doing exercise with a specific focus. For example, Walking around a track with a predetermined heart rate is exercise. Our aim should be directed towards prevention of diseases and to develop a high-level functional capacity, for maintenance of our life force.

Popularly the walking recommended for physical fitness is called 'Fitness Walking'. It is a brisk and aerobic exercise where our heart and lungs work more efficiently to maintain the homeostasis of the body. It improves our cardiovascular and respiratory systems. Les Snowdon in his book 'Fitness Walking' says, "Going aerobics is like changing gear in a car. The body suddenly began to work more efficiently; it runs smoother, burns oxygen more efficiently and we move in to a new dimension".

- Fitness walking uses our both large and small muscle groups, and increases the oxygen demand. It increases the muscle tone and strength. To meet the demand we need to breathe deeply and our heart pumps faster to deliver more blood.

- Fitness walking increases the body's basal metabolic rate (BMR) and burns calories in a tune of approximately 200 calories for every 30 minutes on a plane surface.

- Fitness Walking is safe and prevents injury to joints and muscles due to low impact on them. Our joints become more mobile and strong.

- It isfree, natural, and accessible all the time depending on your free time.

- Fitness walking is a great Stress reliever and makes us feel good. It is the best and the cheapest stress management tool, we have with us.

- Fitness Walking helps us in preserving our lean body mass and decreases our fat mass.

Minimum Duration

We should do Fitness Walking for minimum 25 to 30 minutes a day and five times a week, at our Target Heart Rate. (This is 60 percent to 70 percent of our Maximum Heart Rate).

To Be in Your Target Zone

Speed

We have to start our walking at a slow speed for few days (about a week), with a comfortable pace. We should gradually increase the pace and the time of our fitness walking. The speed to achieve is about 5.5 to 8 km/hour. Better to note down all the progresses in a notebook. This record keeping will keep us motivated and achieve our goal made for the next few months.

$$Speed = Distance/Time$$

For example if we cover 4 kilometres in 30 minutes, the speed will be 4/0.5 hr = 2 km/hour.

Steps Count

In Fitness Walking, the average stride is approximately 2 feet per step. The average steps to cover one mile is around 2640 steps or to cover one kilometre is around 1640 steps.

To customize the personal stride length according to our pedometer, we can measure the distance from toe to toe, or heel to heel, when we take the first stride.

We can calculate the distance by multiplying steps per minute to time spent on walking. For example, if my speed is 150 steps/minutes and I walked for 20 minutes, then

$$\text{Distance covered} = 150 \times 20 = 3000 \text{ steps or 1.8 km or 1.1 miles}$$

Getting Started

- Choose a comfortable shoe.

- Set your exercise goal between health related fitness and sports related fitness.

- We should Start slow and gradually increase our aerobic capacity.

- Let us count our resting pulse rate and measure it until we achieve our Target heart rate. Once we are experienced, we all will be able to keep ourselves within the zone by simply knowing how we feel.

- Warm up body by different set of stretching exercises. Warming up is a useful way to check on how our body feels. We should do it for a minimum of 10 minutes. It increases the circulation to muscles and relaxes our joints.

- We should always take the *longest comfortable stride* for Fitness Walking. Arms should always swing opposite to the feet position and move with the same speed as the leg. For example if our right foot swing forward, our left arm should swing with it.

- In Fitness walking landing of our foot is very important. As we step from one foot to another, the heel of our landing foot should touch the ground first. Once the heel touches the ground, the weight of our body should be shifted forward with the knee bending slightly, rocking on the toes.

- Start walk with a slow speed for about 7 to 10 minutes and gradually reach to a moderate speed and continue for next 20 minutes.

- We should walk with concentration and breathing should be deep. We should not gasp for air and should be able to talk comfortably during brisk walking. If we have any of them then we are overdoing it. In such situations, we should pause for some time and start again. Our heart rate should be at our target heart rate

- We can perceive reaching the target heart rate by following 'Rating of Perceived Exertion', or RPE. Instead of calculating pulse rate frequently, RPE relies more on our gut feelings of how hard we are exercising. When we feel hard during our walking, then probably we are in our aerobic Target zone. RPE runs from six to twenty, where six means no exertion and 20 stars for maximum exertion.

- Once we finished the Fitness Walking, *a cool down period* has to be followed regularly. The pace of our walking has to be reduced over four to five minutes. This reduces the post exercise weakness and sore muscles and helps our heart and respiration to come back to normal.

Walking Pranayama

When we concentrate and breathe deeply during walking, it is considered as walking meditation. When we do it as we take breathing during pranayama, it is known as walking pranayama. It is a better way of combining pranayama while walking.

How We Should Do It

We should walk with head up, shoulders back and chest expanded. Inhale deeply counting from one to three, one count for each step. Then in the retention phase hold the breath until we count one to twelve, each step one count. Then exhale slowly through both nostrils till we count from one to six. This is one cycle. Next, take a pause or rest after one cycle, counting to twelve. This is simple and practical. We can do it anytime and anywhere and at any time.

3. Stress Reduction and Relaxation

We are now living in a world of stress and distraction. We are becoming less tolerant and reactive due to rapid and unplanned industrialization and our fast moving life. From the day we are aware of ourselves, stress has become a companion to us. Education, finance, our family, our work environment, our job insecurities, in some way or the other creates an environment of stress. When these stress persist for a longer period, our heart takes the brunt on it. The stress chemicals adrenaline and cortisol changes the rhythm of our heart. The endothelial damages done by these chemicals lead to thickening of the wall of coronary arteries. Relaxation is the key to reduce stress.

Dr. Dean Ornish in his book writes, "once I made the connection between 'when I felt stressed and why', then stress become my teacher instead of my enemy". Learning to 'let go' and practicing calmness are few of the things advocated in "care for your heart". A proper sleep of 6 to 7 hours relaxes our body.

4. Weight Reduction

Reduction of weight reduces the risk factors associated with heart diseases to a great extent. Due to rapid changes in the socio economic status, there is an increase in obese populations all over the world. Obesity is always associated with high blood pressure, high cholesterol, and diabetes. These groups of people have high level of triglycerides and high LDL. Dietary changes, exercise, strong determination, frequent small diets, low sugar and high fibre intake, high self esteem leads to significant weight loss, which reduces the workload of our heart, pump, resulting in a healthy heart.

5. De Addiction for "Care of Your Heart"

Say No to smoking and minimize the intake of beverage containing caffeine like tea, coffee and soft drinks. Multiple studies have proved that smoking increases the risk of heart disease as nicotine led to clogging of coronary arteries by the formation of clots. This clot formation is due to damage of platelets, alteration of concentration of fibrinogen and blood proteins in the blood. However, the most encouraging fact is that by stopping smoking, we can reduce the chances of heart disease by 50%. The irregular beats or arrhythmia induced by increase intake of caffeine is also reversible.

6. Yoga and Meditation for "Care for Your Heart"

Directly or indirectly, our heart is connected to all the other system of our body. Any activities going on in our body, affect the functioning of our heart to some extent. Heart responds to all external and internal stimuli by two ways. It responds by changing its rhythm to the chemicals secreted by the concerned organ or by gradual narrowing and hardening of coronary arteries causing heart attack. Regular practice of yoga and meditation can reduce the incident of heart attack by calming down our body and mind, resulting in reduction of stress induced damage to our heart. Yoga asana increase the blood circulation and the oxygen carrying capacity of our blood, thus a healthy heart is the by-product. Making simple and small lifestyle changes can bring a great difference to our heart.

Recommendation for Healthy Heart

1. American heart association recommends 30 minutes of moderate to vigorous aerobic exercise every day.

2. Avoid too much high intensity exercise as the study shows increased risk of coronary arterial inflammatory changes.

3. Every exercise session should include a warm up, conditioning phase and cooling down.

4. We should increase our exercising level gradually to reach the target heart rate.

5. Slow and controlled stretching movements to be done until a gentle pull is felt in the muscle concerned. We should hold the stretch for about 20 seconds without pain.

6. We should avoid Extreme cold or hot water bath immediately after exercise.

7. We should keep ourselves hydrated by drinking water before and in between exercise to avoid dehydration.

8. We should stop exercise if we become tired or are short of breath.

9. We should not exercise if not feeling well or during fever.

10. We should stop exercising if our heart beats faster known as palpitation.

11. Doctors should be consulted in case of chest pain.

Chapter VI

Care for Your Gut

"Let's take care of the bacterial ecosystem of our gut, known as microbiota, by taking food which helps them to grow, or else our body is going to react in the same manner as our planet is reacting today by weather changes".

Author

As a general surgeon, I deal with the gut problems mostly. I deal with different groups of people, with different abdominal complain. They come with different symptoms for the same disease. This has made me to go deep into the subject and analyse each one of them in a different manner. Our body gets most of its fuel through this organ and simultaneously it is the organ, which gets abused maximum due to the improper and imbalance food habits. During our medical training, we learned to treat diseases of gut and remove the pathological organ from the body by surgery.

Recent research on gut has unveiled many of the secrets of our gut, which we never thought before. According to a research, our gut accounts for two thirds of our immune system. Gut is the place where the food we eat is absorbed and utilized for energy production. This is the organ, which produces more than 20 different varieties of hormones.

I have often encountered patients with digestive disorders, suffering from depression and irritation. Recent research has linked many of the nervous system disorders to the change in gut microbiota. Our gut is the most neglected organ as compared to other organ as we take it for granted that our gut will manage everything we put inside it.

We view gut as a simple food-processing unit, which just churns the food into a paste with the help of acids and propel it forward to small intestine. The semisolid food then enters the small bowel and nutrients get absorbed from it and passed down to large intestine. In large bowel, the fluid and residual vitamins and mineral get absorbed and the rest of the residual material are then excreted through anus.

For years practicing as a doctor, I had strong faith on this mechanical model of gut but as years passed by, I encountered numerous instances,

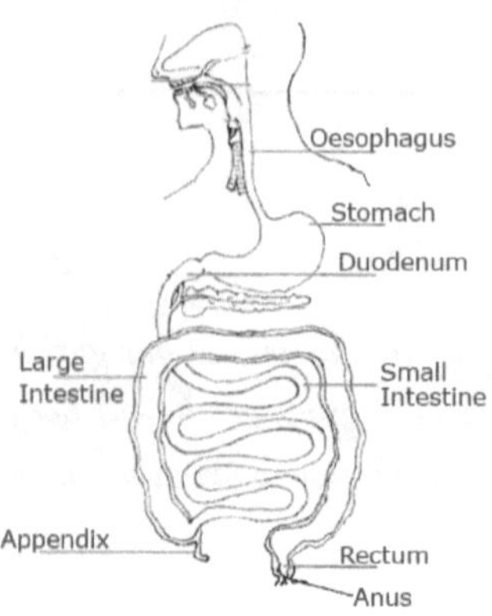

Figure 3

where I could not explain the Patient's complaints with this model. The total modern medicine is centring on this model with numerous drugs and surgical procedures to cure diseases of intestine. My personal experience with milk and milk products made me to ask certain questions to myself.

In my practice as a consultant surgeon, most of my patients visit me for abdominal pain. The most difficult patients to treat are the patients, who used to visit me after consulting many other doctors. When I go through their records, I could see the list of drugs they have already taken. Most of the time, there was no drug left for me to write. In that situation, I always keep the papers aside and start talking to them. I ask about their food habits, their lifestyle, their family and work environment. Then suddenly, in most of the cases, I notice something wrong with their food habits and without even revealing it to them, I ask them to rectify it and give them the same medicines with a different name. To my surprise, most of them recover dramatically. It is the magic of respecting our gut.

Knowing About Our Gut

Before we learn how to take care of our gut, we have to have certain knowledge about our digestive system. We should learn how it controls other systems. Our gut starts with our mouth and ends at our anus.

1. **Mouth** is the beginning of our digestive system and the whole purpose of it is to break the solid food into small pieces and mix the digestive enzyme present in the saliva. This helps in partially digesting the food and easy

passage of food to stomach through oesophagus. Digestive process starts here.

2. **Oesophagus:** Oesophagus is the tube, which carries the food to stomach by series of forward peristaltic movement. It enters the stomach smoothly on the right side of our stomach. Both end of the oesophagus remain closed by muscle spasm to prevent food from regurgitating upward.

3. **Stomach:** Stomach is the place where our food mixed up with the acids and enzymes like pepsin, secreted by the stomach lining. The acid helps to kill the unwanted bacteria, fungi and parasites present in the food we ingest and act on the food materials to break them into its molecular level. The main function of stomach is to churn the food that reaches it, by its peristaltic activity and make them paste like substance called chyme. Many of the water-soluble vitamins and iron gets absorbed from it. The food then passes to duodenum where the bile and pancreatic enzymes mixed with food to break the proteins and fats and carbohydrates. The most interesting event is the stomach lining, is regenerated every two weeks.

4. **Small Intestines:** It is the wonder organ of our body, responsible for the absorption of 90% of the nutrients of the food. It has a surface area, about one hundred times greater than the area of our skin. If we stretch the folding of small intestine, it will be around 7 kilometres. This much large surface area is required to absorb the digested carbohydrates, fat and protein molecules through the walls of small intestine and carry them to liver for further processing. Small intestine, accounts for over 56 percent of intestinal tract but responsible for 90 percent of the calories absorption. The largest masses of immune cells of our body are in our small intestine so it has a large impact on auto immunity. As compared to large intestine, small intestine harbours less bacteria but an imbalance can cause abnormal bowel movement and inflammation sets in the intestinal lining causing leaky gut. Inflammation further kills good bacteria and encourages growth of bad bacteria. Therefore, it is our responsibility to create a good environment for the growth of good bacteria, which further reduces the inflammations of gut. Bacterial overgrowth is a common problem of small intestine due to high carbohydrates diet, known as Small intestinal bacterial overgrowth. This has been linked to many autoimmune

disorders like hypothyroidism, Irritable Bowel syndrome and other conditions like obesity, constipation, bloating etc.

5. **Large Intestine:** Large intestine accounts for 20% of our intestinal length. It is responsible for absorption of food materials, which failed to get absorbed in small intestine. It harbours millions of friendly gut bacteria, which outnumbers cells present in our body. These good gut bacteria form our microbiota. Our microbial ecosystem of our gut plays a great role in our day-to-day life. The food stays in the large colon for about 16 hours or so. The large intestine with its gut flora help us by absorbing important minerals like calcium, fatty acids, vitamin k, vitamin B-12, B-1, B-2 etc which help us in strengthening our, bones, nerves. Once the last useful materials got absorbed from the large intestine, the faecal materials reach the rectum and evacuated from anus. Two circular muscle doors called sphincter controls anus.

Brain-Gut Axis (BGA)

Our gut is the second brain of our body, because of its rich networking of nerve plexus ENS (enteric nerve plexus) and its ability to produce large numbers of neuropeptides, the molecules of information. Enteric nervous system has approximately as many nerves by weight as our entire Central Nervous System, our brain and spine. Neurogastroenterology is a research area, which regards the interaction of central nervous system and the gut- "brain gut axis". Enteric nervous system is a part of peripheral nervous system and a division of autonomic nervous system, which controls the function of gastrointestinal tract. ENS can operate autonomously and communicate with the central nervous system through signals arising from mechanical movements of intestines and by the biological molecules like different enzymes and neurotransmitters and hormones.

The role of BGA is to mediate the environmental effects on gut functions and vice versa. Our gut forms Almost 90 percent of our body's serotonin. Serotonin is the molecule, which plays a major role in our day-to-day activities. Apart from playing an important role in Gut wall movement coordination, it plays a vital role in our sleep, appetite, moods, pain sensitivity and overall well-being.

Our gut produces More than 50 percent of dopamine. Our brain receives the necessary information to act through the production of neuroactive molecules by our gut flora. Any change in our gut flora due to diet, drugs, or disease can change our brain functions. The information flow of Brain Gut Axis is bidirectional and is possible by neural, endocrine, hormonal, and immune links, known as Neuro-immuno-endocrine axis. This communication network is essential for the maintenance of proper gut homeostasis and on our higher cognitive function. Imbalance of Brain gut axis results in many of nervous disorders like, autism, depression, anxiety, irritable bowel syndrome. When we are in stress, the stress hormone, cortisol level increases. This hormone influences the activity of intestinal cells directly resulting in inflammation of the intestinal linings. This leads to leaky gut and damages the gut flora to great extent. These damaged gut flora adversely affect the central nervous system through the neuroendocrine and metabolic pathways.

Gut Ecosystem (Gut Microbiota)

We human beings survive in an ecosystem that is suitable for us and we are in best of our health when our environmental ecosystem is healthy. We have an inbuilt ecosystem where trillions of microscopic organisms live (resides) inside and outside surface of our body. These microscopic organisms in a particular environment are called microbiota. Our large intestine harboured almost 99 percent of the microbiota of our body. Our gut microbiota weighs up to 2 kilos and contains about 100 trillion bacteria. These are the microbes, which break down the undigested food materials of our body, supply the gut with energy, manufactures vitamins, train our immune systems and do the detoxification for our body. We have now started understanding that each one of us have very specific ecosystem and we respond differently to different environment and stimulating factors. Now I have the answer to my question that is why I am intolerant to milk but my father can digest milk easily.

The number of organisms in our microbiota outnumbers our own cells by approximately 10 times. The collective genome of human microbiota is 100 times more than the total genes present in the human being. *The reality is that we are 10 percent human and 90 percent bacteria.* Many studies proved that gut microbiomes in total, plays the role of an organ to the host. Recent research has found different important roles played by our gut microbiota. First, it defends against pathogen colonization by producing antimicrobial substances. It also strengthens the intestinal epithelial barrier to limit bacterial penetration to tissues. It metabolises indigestible food and helps in nutrients absorption. The gut microbiota has an important role in guiding maturation and functionality of host immune system and is critical to peripheral immune education and homeostasis. The gut microbiota composition and activity is influenced by host physiology, diet, immunology, antibiotics use and enteric infection. Disruption of a balanced composition of gut microbiome, termed as **dysbiosis,** may lead to low grade inflammation leading to Irritable Bowel Syndrome [IBS] or Inflammatory Bowel Disease [IBD] and deregulate neuroimmune functions and impacting behaviours.

"Care for your Gut" strongly suggests protecting the environment of our friendly bacteria, which we have been neglecting till date due to our ignorance. It is our responsibility to keep these good bacteria healthy by making their environment optimal.

Foetus inside the uterus is germ free until the child is born. Colonization begins the moment the child, leaves the protective womb environment and is exposed to the mother's birth passage. As the child emerges through it, the child gets a layer of useful coating of bacteria, which forms the first microbiota of its own. The next in line to donate its microbes to the child is the 'breast-feeding' by mother. After this, we get the composition of our gut microbiota from the action we take every day, like licking mother's skin, handling of our environment, the food we eat, our pets etc.

These bacteria are instrumental to the development of other bodily functions like immune functions and our metabolism. The increased incidence of c-section for childbirth has deprived millions of babies from developing their gut flora from mother. This is the cause of increased risk of allergies, asthma, or other immunocompromised conditions. Poor nutrition, use of antibiotics, excessive cleanliness, and too much exposure to bad bacteria are few, which prevent early healthy starting population of the gut. The infant's microbiota resembles the microbiota of an adult as early as 1 year. It has been noticed that with each changes in dietary habit of the infant, there is a significant change in the gut flora and its corresponding microbiome.

The food we eat, our emotional state, our stress level influences the health of our gut microflora. Irrational use of antibiotics and addictions are the major factors for the damage of our gut flora.

The most commonly used tag line of "gut feeling" is an example of how we interpret the effects of stress hormones on our gut,

HUMAN MICROBIOME PROJECT, which gained momentum, few years after the closure of Human genome project (HGP), due to an in depth search for the missing genes. We were expecting around 150000 genes in human being, but we could find only 21000 genes at the end of the HGP. The search for these missing genes completed after the conclusion of HMP in 2012. The study identified that, about 4000 different species of bacteria inhibits in our gut alone and a gene catalogue of 3.3 million genes in the human gut microbiota was found. Individual human are about 99% identically to one another in term of their host genome but are 80-90% different in terms of microbiota of their hand or gut. Recent research is totally directed towards the role of these friendly microbes in our health and diseases.

'Care for your Microbiota' is the need of the time as most of the scientific data now link, many of the dreaded and difficult to treat diseases with the health of the ecosystem of our microbiota. Learning to nurture our microbiota for a better health is a simpler way to living healthy. Following are few steps by which we can help our little friends to grow healthy.

1. Avoid

To get rid of everything that may be damaging it. Avoiding processed food, genetically engineered foods, gluten, fructose helps to stop damaging our gut flora. Judicious use of antibiotics, antimicrobial soaps and cleaning agents prevents the microbiota damage. We should avoid dairy foods.

2. Ingest

Eating for the growth of microbiota is the simplest way to care for your gut. Low carbohydrates, high Fibre and moderate fats should be the goal. Complex carbohydrates found in vegetables, nuts, beans are the best choice. We should avoid or minimize processed foods, candy, baked goods, and fruit juices. Egg protein is a good choice. Dark chocolate base can be a great alternate sweet dish.

3. Include Pre and Probiotic

Probiotics are fermented foods that contain healthy live bacteria and yeasts. These bacteria resist bad bacteria, lower inflammation, helps to absorb important nutrients and vitamins. These provide antibiotics, antiviral and antifungal coverage. These include fermented foods like yogurts, pickles, fermented rice, fish, soy sauces, buttermilk etc.

Prebiotics are food, which the gut bacteria eat to survive and are mostly indigestible fibres that we eat. The more we give them this feed, the stronger they will become and the healthier we will be. Onion, garlic, raw wheat barn, backed wheat flour, banana, broccoli, lemons, oats, carrots, honey, dark leafy vegetables are few commonly used prebiotics. Recommendation is to consume 5 grams of prebiotic food per day.

4. Lifestyle and Environmental Change

This includes few simple day-to-day, regular activities and preventive measures, which can keep our microbiota healthy and help us to enjoy life. **SMOKING** causes a great damage to our bacterial population. Avoidance of active and passive smoking can help us to rebuild our damaged gut flora. **AIR POLLUTION** alters our microbiota. Regular use of air filters can minimize the damage. Water filters, indoor plants, saying no to chemical skin care products are few measures to escape from the environmental damage to bacterial flora. **EXPOSURE** to sun can be of immense help to our microbiota and lots of research now proved that sun exposure prevents cancers by helping the normal commensalism to grow. Spending more time with **NATURE** improves the bacterial diversity in human beings. Living closure to agricultural land, exposure to pets, well-ventilated house expose us to microbes, which tone our immune system. **REGULAR EXERCISE** improves our internal environment and helps in the growth of our friendly bacteria. Hormones like noradrenalin help the growth of healthy bacteria. Exercise induces noradrenalin.

5. Sleep

Sleep is necessary for the re growth of the damaged bacterial flora. Good sleep is equivalent to good internal environment. An adequate sleep of six hrs is good for our microbiota and our health.

6. Stress

Stress affects our gut and its microbiota negatively. Researchers all over the world have documented the negative impact of stress hormones on gut mucosa and the microbiota. Stress hormones fuel the growth of dangerous bacteria.

Stress reduction by deep breathing, meditation and exercise, decreases the damage caused by stress. Probiotics has shown significant reduction in stress in individuals. Making new friends, finding the purpose of living, spending time with loved ones, avoiding too much of TV and internet are few things we can adopt reduce our stress and strengthen our microbiota.

Care for Your Leaky Gut

Leaky gut is a condition, when there is an increased intestinal permeability to gut bacteria and toxins to circulation, causing different abdominal symptoms.

Some of the conditions which contribute to leaky gut include, use of painkillers for a longer time, pathogenic bacteria, alcohol, dysbiosis, chronic stress, hormonal imbalance etc.

Symptoms includes, bloating of abdomen, food sensitivities, chronic diarrhoea, skin rashes, chronic joint pain, peripheral neuropathy pain, Alzheimer's, anxiety etc.

1. Identifying and removing the factors responsible for leaky gut. It is better to avoid painkillers, alcohol, smoking, and remove gluten-containing grains like wheat from the diet and managing stress. We should exclude refined sugar, dairy products from our diet.

2. Our food should be replaced with gut friendly food, which will rebuild the gut lining. We recommend eating wholesome food, increasing omega 3 fatty acids, high fibre diets and amino acid supplements.

3. Eating fermented food containing pre and probiotics will replace the gut microbiota.

4. Low carbohydrate diet starves the bacteria, which can reduce bacterial overgrowth.

5. Eat a fresh and ripe fruit at a time, in empty stomach. Fruits low in sugar like, apple, banana, grapefruit, kiwis, berries.

6. Green leafy Vegetables like fresh herbs, sprouts and radish, peas, mushrooms, cauliflower are to be included in the food.

7. Sleep for 6 to 8 hours to give proper rest to the body.

8. It is important to eliminate the infection or overgrowth of bad bacteria by appropriate drugs.

Chapter VII

Care for Your Mind

The power to lead a Healthy life forever is always within our reach. Only need is to align ourselves into that mode. A burning desire, self-commitment, a learning mindset and an attitude of self-love will lead us there comfortably.

Author

Twenty years back, when I started my practice as surgeon, one incident had turned my focus toward the power of mind. One evening, I did attend a patient in casualty, who was on the verge of death. His son, breaking a train journey, brought MR. B to my hospital. He was on way to his home after being refused by a reputed hospital, for treatment. Mr. B had a huge pancreatic tumour, which was obstructing his stomach and bile duct, causing jaundice. His bilirubin level was 37 mg. He had few liver nodes by then. His vital sign were poor. When I first examined him, I thought he would never see the next day. I was about to talk to his family regarding the prognosis of Mr. B, suddenly he caught hold my hand and started looking to me with a great expectation and hope. Very slowly, he uttered two lines. 'Doctor please operate on me, I want few more days to live for my younger son'. I do not know until date, what made me decide that day, to do a palliative surgery on Mr. B, knowing very well, patient may die during operation. Retrospectively now I can tell, it was his will to live and the faith on himself, which was the main driving force behind that decision. Next day I did a Triple bypass surgery on Mr. B, to divert

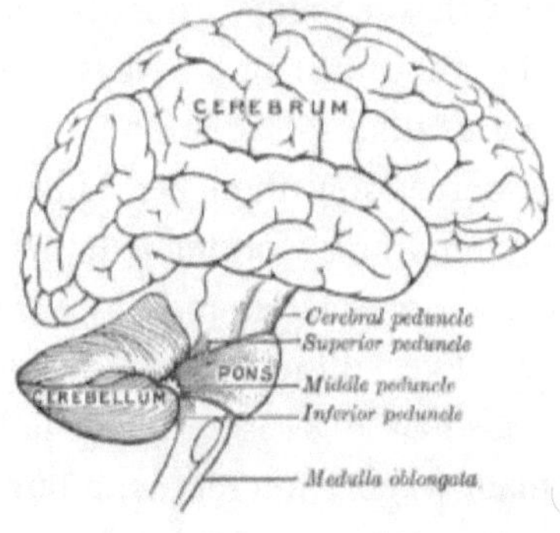

bile and food through other opening. To my surprise, he recovered well from anaesthesia and postoperative period was smooth. On third day, the bilirubin level had come down to 23 and on ninth postoperative day, it was 4 mg. I discharged him on 12th day and was on normal diet. I was happy that, now MR. B could eat, till he die as the expected survival for this type of stage IV cancer is maximum 6 months. Mr. B left the hospital with a promise to be back for a follow up after a week. This case made me to think weather; I should give the credit for the success of this surgery to me, for my surgical skill, or to the patient for his dynamic will power to survive the episode.

Mr. B never came back to me after that day for any type of complaint or follow up, until one afternoon 4 years after discharge. I had almost forgotten him, but when he narrated the surgery, I could remember him. This time the scenario was different. He was depressed, sick and weak. That day he told me the truth. During last four year, he did help his son to be self-sufficient and now both of his children abandoned him with a servant. He asked me to hospitalize him till death. To my surprise and in spite of my medical care he died 10 days after the incident. This made me to realize the power of mind. Mr. B could survive for 4 years with a huge tumour with liver metastasis by his will power and died the moment he lost it.

When I started looking at my patients through this mindset, I observed many more deviations, from the expected ways of recover. I started noticing the recovery period of few patients faster than other did. The pain perception is totally different for different patients. Then I made it a routine to give postoperative pain injections on demand only. To my surprise, the requirements of analgesic reduced by 50 to 60%. These observations made me to go deeper in to the subject of role of our mind over our body.

Medical research now has enough evidences about the relationship between the body and the mind. Our mind plays a mysterious role to keep us healthy or drift us towards illness. Our mind is a set of cognitive faculties including consciousness, perception, thoughts, judgment and memories. In fact, it is our thoughts and emotions working together as one unit, which we call mind. We are different from other animals by our power of thinking and the behaviour that follows. Everything we do to survive in this world has a biological basis, in the sense that, it is associated or linked with the biological process or events. The main way we interact with our world is the sensation we receive through our five senses. Sensation leads to perception and our perception create our thoughts. Thought leads to emotions and ultimately results in our behaviour.

Our brain is the entity where the information we perceived by our five senses are processed, analyzed and sent to the necessary organs for implementation. The main concern of our brain is self-preservation and preservation of the species. We should have the basic knowledge about how our brain functions and how can we have a control over it to direct it for our own benefit.

Just think of an event, which happened around you. You are reading a newspaper, and suddenly you smell of something burning, next reaction will be you jump from your couch and start searching for the source and you are on your toes till you find the source and take the appropriate measures. Now the question is, how the mare information of smell, triggers your emotions and the behaviour that followed it. The answer is the activity of Neurons: cells that are specialized for the task of receiving, analyzing and processing information.

Neurons are the building blocks of our nervous system, a complex network that regulates our bodily functions. Our nervous system, though functions as an integrated whole, it is often viewed as two major portions. The **central nervous system** consisting of brain and spinal cord and the **peripheral nervous system** consists of the somatic and autonomic nervous system. It is the autonomic nervous system, which controls the internal organs, glands and muscles, over which we have, no or little voluntary control plays a major role in our health.

Dr. Candace Pert, a neuropharmacologist in 1970 found the receptors for opiates, while working for her doctoral thesis at John Hopkins School of medicine. Dr. Pert's discovery of receptors on cell wall started a new revolution that created a paradigm shift within the field of medicine. Further research on hypothesis helped to create, the foundation of an entirely new interdisciplinary branch of medicine called "Psychoneuroimmunology" (PNI). Dr. Pert's research provided scientific evidence that a biochemical basis for awareness and consciousness exist and our body and mind are one. Out thought and emotions are the bridges that link the two.

Our brain is a three-pound mass of fatty tissue and behaves like a supercomputer. This single organ controls our all body activities, ranging from our emotions, learning, Memories, Our heart rate, our respiration, our sexual behaviour etc. everything we do and think and feel is controlled by how our brain cells or neurons connects to one another. These connections are like wiring of an electrical circuit. So continuously, we are wired or rewired, depending on the firing of the neurons, as a result of stimulus generated by our immediate environment. Therefore, it is all about communication between one hundred billion of brain cells with trillions of other body cells, through hundreds of chemicals, that shapes our thoughts, actions and behaviour. Our prefrontal cortex is our thinking brain. In reality, our brain is not running the show from our head, but the intelligent biological molecules distribute throughout our body runs the show by constantly sending and receiving the information.

Brain Waves

Our behaviours and emotions are nothing but the communication between neurons within our brain. We produce Brain waves by the synchronised electrical pulses from mass of neurons communicating with each other. Our brain wave changes according to the state of our activities and feelings. Brain waves are measured in Hertz (cycles / minutes)

Brain waves	Frequency Hertz	Implications
Delta waves	0.5 to 3 HZ	Found in deep meditation and sleep. Healing and regeneration are stimulated in this state. This is the reason we need deep restorative sleep.
Theta wave	4 to 7 Hertz	Found in sleep and deep meditation. Our senses are withdrawn from the external world and focus on signals from within.
Alpha waves	8 to 14 Hertz	This is the most harmonious brain wave. Dominate during meditative state. This is the resting state of brain and 'the power of now'
Beta waves	14 to 38 Hertz	Beta brain waves dominate our normal waking state of consciousness. Beta activity is present when we are alert, attentive, engaged in problem solving, judgment, decision making, or focused mental activity.

When we meditate, we reduce our brain wave frequency to alpha. This is the level where we harness the power of subconscious mind maximally. Feelings of intuition, creative ideas, inspiration thoughts and ideas come to us while we are in the alpha state (Jose Silva). Going to Alpha frequency is good to reprogram our mind. We can overcome many bad habits, stress and program our mind for goal settings to reach our dreams in alpha state.

Anatomy of Brain

Anatomically we divide our brain mainly into three basic units, the forebrain, the midbrain and the hindbrain.

The forebrain is the largest and highly developed part of human brain. It consists of cerebrum and the structures of inner brain thalamus, hypothalamus and hippocampus. It is the source of our intellectual activities. It is the site of our memories and enables us to think and plan. It divides into two halves, by a deep fissure that communicates with each other through a track of thick nerve fibres. The expression of self-consciousness is specifically associated with our prefrontal cortex. This enables us to realise our personal identity and helps us in our decision-making and future planning.

The midbrain controls our reflexes and is part of the circuit responsible for voluntary action.

The hindbrain consists of our brain stem and cerebellum. It controls our vital functions such as our heart and respiration. Cerebellum is responsible for our gait and balancing of our body.

Left side of our brain is logical and rational. It is responsible for sequential and linear mode of thought. It is associated with competitiveness, aggression and selfishness. Left hemisphere of our brain is responsible for Verbal communication, reading, writing and talking.

Right side of brain is very imaginative, artistic, intuitive and psychic. It has association with feminine qualities of love, compassions and nurturing. It deals with our perception and concept formation. It creates pictures of the perceived information. It is creative and has three-dimensional perceptions.

Perceptions

Perception is the ability to see, hear, smell, touch or tastes something through our senses. It is impossible for us to be aware of, every information, which reaches to our brain through five senses. We only perceive those objects and events that have meaning to us. Therefore, perception is the identification, interpretation and organisation of events occurring in our immediate environment. The things we perceive mostly depend on our past memories and the moods and feelings associated with it. The event, which we perceive as good when we are happy, can be, interpreted just the opposite when we are in a bad mood. We differ in the way we perceive an event, depending on our own way of looking through it. Taking care of the way we look into an event by overcoming our own memories, preconceptions, attitude and blockage; we can lead a healthy life forever.

There are three sources of perceptions. The first one is the most primitive, which we acquire through our genome. These are fundamental reflex behaviours or we call them instincts and are natural. The second source of our perception is our life experiences stored in our subconscious mind. Finally, the third source of our perception is from our self-conscious mind of creative imagination. Here we perceive the things, which are not real, but our mind considers them 'as if' it is already there.

Thought

When our senses perceive stimulus from the environment, our mind receive it after a lot of deletion and distortion of the information. When our brain processes the information and gives it a meaning, it becomes a Thought. Thought leads us to feelings and helps in our decisions making. In lower animals, it is the instinct, which does the work, but in human being, our thoughts can dominate our thinking, emotions and behaviour, unless we outgrow it. A mere thought of illness, changes our behaviour and opens up the ways to sickness.

Emotions

Emotion is nothing but the state of a person, at a particular moment of life. These are the personal feeling such as anger, joy, love, hate, sorrow, disgust, acceptance, anticipation, surprise etc. Our emotions are the results of our thoughts or directly created from our memories. Our emotions have a greater role on our health as they bring changes in our body by altering the chemical and physiological composition of our body. For example, when we are in fear our body goes to fight or flight mode and the chemical adrenalin pumped in to our circulation causing increase in heart rate, redirection of blood to peripheral circulation for immediate action. Similarly, when we are in love, our body produces oxytocin, which relaxes us. Recent research has enough proof that integration of the brain with our body is at a molecular level. These molecules of emotions have two components.

1. Receptors
2. Peptides

Receptors sit on the surface of our cell wall and are present in hundreds of thousands on average cells. Specialized cells such as Neurons might have millions of receptors surroundings them. These receptors act as tiny scanners and sensors, which wait patiently until an exact chemical key comes along, that, will fit into them. These chemical keys are "LEGANDS".

LEGANDS are of three types: neurotransmitters, steroids and peptides.

Neurotransmitters are the smallest, simplest molecules manufactured in the brain to transmit information between neurons.

Steroids, including sex hormones testosterone, progesterone and estrogens, starts out as cholesterol and by a series of chemical steps transforms into a specific type of hormones.

Peptides account 95 percent of LEGANDS. Our body produces these LEGANDS, all over and deliver its chemical message to cell receptors and transmit its message deep into the cells. Once produced, they trigger chains of biochemical reactions, which can bring huge changes within our cells, either positive or negative one. Following are few important molecules of our emotions and health.

"Care for your mind", necessitate each individual to know little about these *biological molecules,* which governs our mind and body.

1. Adrenalin

This is the body's stress chemicals. It triggers body's fight or flight response. Once our mind perceives a stressful situation, our body prepares itself to face it or escape from it. This causes our air passages to expand, so that more oxygen can diffuse into circulation, to supply the demand of our muscles. This helps us get the strength to fight the danger or flee. It also triggers our blood vessels to contract and redirect the blood flow towards major muscle groups and to our heart and lungs. This is the reason we can do extraordinary physical strength when we are in danger. After the stressful situation is over, the effects remain up to an hour.

Sometime the body will release the hormone when it is in stress but actually, it is not in real danger. In this type of situation, the person feels dizziness, light-headedness and hazy vision due to the less blood supply to these organs. The extra glucose released, in fight or flight response for immediate energy, remain inside the body with no purpose to serve. This causes the person restless and irritable. Excessive high level of these chemical due to stress without real danger can cause heart damage, nervousness and sleeplessness, stomach ulceration, indigestion and gut imbalance.

2. Dopamine

Dopamine is an addictive and feel good chemical, involved in reinforcing behaviour. For example, if you do something, that your brain is programmed to, like drinking tea just after getting up from bed in the morning to feel fresh. This activity releases a small dose of dopamine as soon as you get up and drink the tea. This you may not feel or be aware of but wherever you are, your mind will crave for the tea the moment you get up.

Dopamine's main function is to activate pleasures and rewards, mood fixation, attention, memory improvement. A balanced proportion of this chemical in our body keeps us inspired, motivated, satisfied and makes us feel great.

This is the reason why it is advisable to break down big goals into small pieces. This will create series of little finish line, which will release dopamine, every time we reach the target. This will create a constant dopamine flow in our body. We can always get a dopamine hit, if we reward ourselves by gifting something we want, or visit a restaurant whenever we complete a small task. Foods rich in tyrosine, one of the main components of dopamine, can give our body a little nudge to produce this happy chemical. Cheese, spirulina, soy foods, seafood, chicken and turkey, nuts and seeds, eggs, beans are rich in tyrosine.

3. Serotonin

Serotonin is the happy chemical of the body. It is flow increase whenever we feel significant and important. The moment someone gives importance to us, we feel happy and ready to serve him or her. People fall into gangs and criminal activity because that culture facilitates serotonin production. The opposite is also true, that is when we feel depressed, and our serotonin level is low. Walnuts, Pineapple, banana, kiwis, and tomatoes are few things, which increase our serotonin level.

4. Endorphins

Endorphin is the chemical for our survival and is responsible for the evolution of human beings to the present age. This is responsible for the "runners high", so that runners feel good while performing better as endorphin masks the pain. These chemicals activate the pain receptors, causing the analgesic effect. This is the reason behind our smooth performance of a job, in spite of their toughness.

There are certain foods like chocolate, strawberries, orange, spicy food; Ginseng etc that stimulates endorphins production in the body.

5. Oxytocin

Oxytocin is a chemical of love, trust, intimacy and healthy relationships. Both men and women release it during orgasm and by mother during childbirth and breastfeeding. This chemical increases fidelity, and the cultivation of Oxytocin is essential for creating strong bonds and improved social interactions.

The simplest way to keep Oxytocin flowing is to give someone a hug. Dr. Paul Zak explains that interpersonal touch not only raises levels of Oxytocin, but also reduces cardiovascular stress and improves immunity. The moment I touch my patients while examining or counselling, I can see the stress, vanishing from their face. We can always feel when someone receives a gift; his or her Oxytocin level rises unexpectedly.

Behaviour

Behaviour is the response of an individual to an action, environment, person or a stimulus. In the human, the behaviour can be anywhere from physical action, verbal response to body language. Our resulting behaviours decide the state of our mind. We always have choices to behave differently, to a particular stimulus. When we behave in a particular way to a certain stimulus, then it becomes a habit and we respond in a habitual way. We may remain calm and flood our circulation with serotonin or react to the same event and bring adrenaline rush into our circulation. Consciously helping the body to produce the above biological molecules in our body, we can change our behaviours. Our subconscious mind controls most our behaviours.

Our behaviours are solely responsible for the actions we take to survive in this world and decide the state of our health. With the help of the knowledge we gain, about the natural pharmacopoeia potentially present within our body, we can literally dictate our health conditions.

Conscious and Subconscious Mind

Throughout our life, we have been told that our mind plays an important role in our health. We have to understand certain things about it very clearly. According to Dr. Joseph Murphy, our mind possesses two distinctive characteristics and we live in a duality. We call them conscious and subconscious mind. The conscious mind is the voluntary mind and the subconscious mind the involuntary mind. Our subconscious mind controls Ninety-five percent of our behaviour and functioning of our body. Subconscious mind take the reasoning of the conscious mind, as command and execute it. Our subconscious mind does not discriminate between positive or negative, right or wrong, good or bad. It is as if our mind is a garden and we are the gardener, then we are planting seeds of conscious thoughts in our subconscious mind throughout out the day by our habitual thinking. As we sow in our subconscious mind, so shall we reap in our body and mind.

Our subconscious mind is a powerful data processor and it stores massive amount of data from the direct and indirect learning experiences of our life. As an information processor, our subconscious mind is one million times more powerful than our conscious mind. Our conscious mind allows us to assess and respond to the tasks present at that point of time, in our environment. Our subconscious mind operates without our knowledge, most of the time and plays a greater role in our decision making process. If we go by the principle of cause and effect, *every thought is a cause and our health is an effect*. Therefore, it is necessary to take charge of our thoughts to bring forth the desirable health for ourselves. If we repeatedly present the picture of good health consciously, then the subconscious mind produces the same in reality.

A very important aspect of 'Care for our mind' includes, the management of our stress and emotions so that, they will not affect our brain and our physical body. Every one of us, pass through many stressful situations every day and we are aware of the need to control our stress. To some extent, we need the stress mechanism to run in our body, to give us protection from dangers and to achieve something bigger. It is an adaptive response. Somehow, many a times, we fail to take the corrective measures to balance it properly. It is our lack of management of our own life properly; we become a victim of illness.

What Happens to Our Body When We Are in Stress?

This is a million dollar question. To know this we have to go through the mechanism by which our body responds to a situation. When we perceive an event which is emotionally disturbing, life threatening or as an impending unfavourable situation, our body goes into a different physiological state. We call it fight or flight response as explained previously. Our ancestors use to utilise this physiological state for their benefit because of their hard work and survival. In this fast moving world these physiological changes becomes a burden to the body and behave like a wild animal. Uncontrolled and without any purpose, it destroys our health little by little every day.

Though there are many ways of getting over the stress, but the most important is the recognition of the stressors and the awareness in ourselves that we are stressing ourselves to the limits of harming ourselves. It is beyond the scope of the book to go details but we will have enough ways to manage it.

'Care for Your Health' advocate, management of Stress by the following S.T.R.E.S.S. Formula.

- **S – Self-love for self-growth**
- **T – Taming our mind**
- **R – Recognition of the stressors**
- **E – Exercise without excuse**
- **S – Sleep adequately**
- **S – Simplification of life matters**

S — Self Love for Self-Growth

One of the common causes of our stress is, not in recognising one's self worth. Self worth is just another word to explain self-love. Self-love means thinking of our self first, thinking of our own well-being first and to be proud of ourselves. It means, putting your needs before others, at a time when others need you. It is like learning to release the brakes; you have been putting on your life since long.

Anita Moorjani, a woman with a history of near death experience, after a prolonged suffering from an end stage cancer disease, mentioned very nicely about self-love. In her book "Dying to be me", she wrote about the importance of self-love in our life. The moment she had gone into the NDE (near death experience), she was in a place, where there was no time and space reality. She asked herself a question in that moment of her life. Why I have to suffer so much? During that NDE period, she had a revelation and the answer came to her. She suddenly realised that she had never loved herself. The whole life she wasted, on convincing people that she loved everyone. According to her, the bitter truth is we always pretend to love people close to us, but forget to love ourselves. This creates a big barrier for our mind to move freely and with time, it becomes worse and kills the fighting spirit inside us. Ultimately, it leads to ill health and suffering.

The best way for loving self, is to practice "**ME FIRST**". Your need rather than your want should come first. Caring for your body should take the centre stage in the form of regular exercise and good food habits. We have to become liberal to our mistakes. We should forgive and forget those incidents, which are the main cause of our pain and agony. We have to create a personal space to live our own life, as we are the creator of our good health.

T – Taming the Mind Through Meditation, Prayers, Visualisation and Affirmations, Autogenic Relaxation

There is a saying, that it is not the stress, which causes damages to our body, but the chemicals it generates during that period. It is how we perceive the stress: that causes more harm or good to our health. We are in a world, where we have to face stressful situations every moment of our life. If by any means we can prevent the stressful situations to enter into our mind, then we will be able to prevent the damage to happen in our body. There are many ancient but practical methods, which are time proved, help us to tame our mind so that stress can cause minimal damage to our body. Meditation, affirmations, visualisation, prayers helps us to prevent the ongoing damage to our body by these chemicals.

A. Meditation

Meditation or dhyana is the seventh of eight-fold path of yoga and it follows dharana or concentration. It refers to a state in which the body is consciously relaxed and the mind becomes calm and focused. It is a practice when an individual uses the technique of mindfulness of focusing their mind on an object, thought or activity to train attention and awareness to achieve a mentally clear and emotionally calm state.

The purpose of meditation varies widely. We should do it for simple relaxation, to get away from hectic stressful situations, or to communicate with God to get enlightenment. It is a way to balance a person's physical, mental and emotional health.

We are living in a world full of distractions and every moment our mind faces information overload. Based on the information we receive and process it in our mind, we react to the situations and subject our body to stress and restlessness. Meditation may simply serve as a mean of relaxation method, to bring the body and mind back to normal state.

We have to learn a little about the benefits of meditation. These are few benefits of doing meditation on a regular basis.

1. Meditation subjects our body into deep rest, by decreasing the metabolic rate, slowing our heart rate, and reducing the load of the heart.

2. Meditation lowers the level of stress hormone adrenaline and cortisol, by increasing the parasympathetic activities.

3. It reduces the blood cholesterol level.

4. It has an anti-aging effect on the body and mind.

5. Meditation Increases the immunity of the body.

6. Meditation Improves learning ability, memory and our cognitive functions.

7. It Acts as an antidepressant and anti anxiety activity.

8. It Increases our emotional intelligence.

9. In chronic lifestyle diseases, it improves the quality of life largely.

10. Meditation is of great help during drugs de-addiction programs.

11. It balances the activity of two hemispheres, leading to better coordination, calmness and brings better equilibrium in life.

The '*Care for your health*' program advocates sparing of 30 to 45 minutes every day for meditation. We can learn meditation from trained teachers or through guided meditation recordings. A person can choose any one technique of meditations and do it sincerely. Meditation can be "concentrative" where we focus on a specific object, word, mantras, or mindfulness where our focus is on the background perceptions. We all should be aware of the basic know how of meditation, which can be upgraded to higher versions with experience.

Three basic needs for meditation are:

1. A quiet space
2. Comfortable posture
3. A positive attitude

We can start meditating, by choosing a quiet space and a comfortable sitting posture. We can do it by sitting on the floor or sitting on a chair. The spine has to be straight and in a line with the head. Let us start with few deep relaxing breathing by closing our eyes. Now let us concentrate on a sound or word (a mantra), or visualise a peaceful environment or on an image. By doing this our mind will drift away from unwanted thoughts and will calm down. We have to do it for a minimum of 30 to 35 minutes regularly to get the benefits of meditation.

B. Visualisation

Visualisation is a method by which we create a mental image of something we want from our life. This is not a new thing, as unconsciously we always create the image of the things, before we receive them in our life. It is an everyday affair, which goes unnoticed mostly. It is our natural power of imagination. Someone has rightly said, "Wherever we are today, it's because of the thought and images we have of ourselves, in our mind today and we can change our future by just changing our thoughts and images". Most of our suffering is because of living a life of what we see around us. We are living in a disease conscious world, where we are always trying not to fall ill. By this, we attract illness, as image of illness is in our mind.

Visualisation is a great tool to reduce our stress and to lead a healthy life. Visualisation is a tool through which our mind can communicate with our body. The images we create in our mind act as a signal to our body and prepare it for a transformation. In reality, our brain does not know the difference, between what is real and what is imaginary. Its only job is to process the signals and create new neuronal connections. Once the brain cells trained according to a particular way, it performs only in that particular way. Once we visualise ourselves in a peaceful, calm and healthy human being, our body will follow the direction of our mind.

Shakti Gawain, in her bestselling book, "Creative Visualisation", mentioned four basic steps for visualisation. We have to,

- First, set a goal of what we want to achieve. This may be to remain healthy throughout, to lead a peaceful life, to get rid of pain etc.

- Secondly, we have to create a mental picture of that state of healthy life or the feelings of peaceful or no suffering state of mind.

- Thirdly start focusing on that mental picture during meditation or all throughout the day.

- Lastly be positive about the outcome. See yourself or feel that you have already achieved it.

For example, we are visualising for a healthy heart, we have to follow the following steps. First, we have to choose a quiet place and sit on a chair or on the floor, keeping our spine and head straight. Than with deep abdominal breathing, the whole body has to be relaxed. With every inhalation, let us visualise our heart beating rhythmically, with a rate of 72 beats per minute. We can visualise the heart contracting and relaxing with each inhalation and exhalation respectfully. We can see the colour of our heart changing to red while contracting, due to 100% flow of blood to heart muscle. We can visualise the four main vessels supplying to heart muscles, intact and free from any blockage. We can also have the feel of blood reaching to all the cells of our body due to wonderful pumping action of our Heart. This need deep concentration and regular practice.

C. Prayers

"Man's need for prayer is as great as his need for bread. As food is necessary for the body, prayer is necessary for the soul. I have not a shadow of doubt that the strife and quarrels with which our atmosphere is so full today are due to the absence of the spirit of true prayer. True prayer never goes unanswered. When the mind is full of prayerful thoughts, everything in the world seems to be good and agreeable. Prayer is essential for progress of life".

—Mahatma Gandhi—

Prayer is a great stress reducer for human beings. Research shows that people who are more religious or spiritual can cope with stress better than non-religious persons can. People who do pray regularly, heals faster from illness and remain healthy. Dr. Roberta lee, in her book *"The Super Stress Solution"* has mentioned the benefit of prayer on our health and healing. People, who pray passionately and with an intention of positive outcome, recover faster from illness and maintain a healthy life until death. We can pray vocally or we can pray during meditation for a positive outcome. When we pray, we pass on the burden, for a short period, to higher self. Our mind becomes peaceful and our attitude towards the stressors becomes less reactive.

According to Sri Ramakrishna, the prerequisites of prayer are faith, absence of ego, spirit of sacrifices and firm believe in the higher self. During prayer we have to open up our heart and mind before the omnipresent, whatever it may cost us. Prayer is self-suggestion, in which we are instructing our subconscious mind to change things for better.

My Experience

I personally pray to God, every time I start my day. In front of my consulting table, an old plaque is hanging since last 25 years, which read as follows,

"Dear God...

Please take my hand and guide them.

Grant me the strength to help my patients and their families.

The skill to ease their sufferings.

The understanding to diagnose their needs.

The kindness of heart to care for them and reassure their fears.

Please be beside me every day, as I rely on you

The greatest of all healers...

Amen..."

The moment I read this prayer, I feel myself charged and get ready for the day. I could see my physiology changing, my posture and my behaviour changing and I become more empathetic towards my patients. During surgery, many a time I was stuck in situations, where I did not know how to proceed next. When I am in such situation, I just ask my assistant to stop for a moment and we pack the wound. I pray God for two minutes to show me the path. To my surprise, after two minutes of wait, when we start the operation, everything becomes smooth and easy sailing as before. This has happened so many times that, nowadays my assistants ask me to take a break and pray, whenever we are in similar situation.

Prayer for Health

To pray for a healthy life, we have to choose a quiet place, and take few deep breathing as described in 'care for your breath' chapter. Now Let us ask God for a beautiful and healthy body and Visualise ourselves in a great state of health and mind with all of our organs functioning absolutely in harmony with nature. We should thank God for protecting us from all the offenders to our body. Now during prayers we should feel the healthy and strong body we already have. We can see a healing light gradually encircling us, dissolving all our stress, and suffering with it. After 3 to 5 minutes of prayer, gradually open your eyes and relax with an anticipation of God listening to your prayer.

D. Affirmations

Affirmations are positive statements that can help to change and overcome our self-sabotaging and negative thoughts. These are statements, used to reprogram the subconscious mind and when said repeatedly with emotion, influences the mind and manifests changes in life. We should repeat affirmations again and again verbally, mentally or by writing down. When worded correctly, positively with emotions, affirmations can tap into unlimited creative power of our subconscious mind. Self-affirmations help to mitigate the effect of stress. As physical exercise is for physical health, the affirmations are exercises of our mind for our mental health. Studies have proved that short affirmation exercise; boost the problem solving ability of chronically stressed people. Affirmations are most effective when used along with visualisation.

Rules for Affirmations

1. Affirmations are to be stated in present tense.
2. Affirmations should be in positive statements.
3. Affirmations should be short and specific.
4. Affirmations should be credible and achievable.

5. Affirmations should be repeated with emotions and one should be persistent.

Examples:

1. I am now perfectly healthy in body mind and spirit.
2. I love and accept myself exactly as I am.
3. I am at peace.
4. I am doing my work effortlessly.
5. I am the best person for the job assigned to me
6. My ability is greater than any challenges I have to face.
7. I am inundated with joy, enthusiasm and bliss.
8. I use my fear and anger to fuel in me courage and determination
9. I am committed to live my life with passion.
10. I bring out the best in others.
11. I am supremely happy now.

E. Autogenic Relaxation

Autogenic relaxation is a technique by which the relaxation response of our body is, obtained by conscious command to a particular organ by self-suggestions. Dr. J H. Schultz, a German psychiatrist, popularized this method. Autogenic relaxation involves repetition of a set of visualizations that induces a state of relaxations of a particular group of muscle. We can transform ourselves into a relaxed state through our power of thoughts. We can also train our mind to respond to a specific event by programming through guiding principles.

This technique works properly by practicing regularly after proper training. Through autogenic relaxation training, we program our subconscious mind to our advantage, which is responsible for 90 percent of our activities. We can program our subconscious through our visual images, through our thought process and by the kinaesthetic or feelings.

How to Do It

We should do Autogenic training, in any relaxed position like sitting, horizontal sleeping or reclined position. Repeatedly verbal commands are given to a particular limb or organ to relax. For example, commands are given to feel heavy or become warm. Here patience is a virtue. We have to repeat each command multiple times, until we reach the required relaxation state. We call the commands given as 'formula' in Autogenic Training. Whenever a formula is applied to a part, body gradually starts following it and in time, it goes into autopilot mode.

R — Recognition of the Stressors

Stressors are events or conditions in our surrounding that trigger stress.

Stress can result from anything that annoys us, excites us, threatens us, worries us, hurries us, anger us, frustrates us or challenges us. The sources of stress are mainly three.

1. Situational Stressors

It is due to stressors present in our immediate environment. Our job environment, family circumstances, noise pollution, excessive or inadequate light in workplace, overcrowding, heavy traffic, long working hours etc are few among them.

2. Body Stress or Physiological Stressors

These are stressors, which put strain on our body. It may be conditions like, very hot or cold climate, chronic illness, injuries, pain, addictions, etc.

3. Mental Stressors

Psychological stressors are negative perception of life events or situations. Few of the examples are depression, divorce, debt, our emotions, dealing with difficult boss, our relationship, unrealistic expectations, perfectionism, pessimism etc.

Remember it is not the stressors, but the way we perceive the stressors through our five senses is important.

E — Exercise Without Excuse

People follow this most common stress booster with or without their knowledge. This not only improves our health, it also relaxes our tense muscles and induces sleep. When we Exercise regularly, it improves the blood flow to our brain, resulting in better oxygenation of brain tissue. Exercise pumps up the chemical endorphins, our feel good neurotransmitter in to our circulation and suppress the stress hormone adrenaline and cortisol. Endorphin is a natural painkiller and induces sleep resulting in stress reduction.

S — Sleep Adequately

Sleep is a natural state of our body and mind when our neurological, muscular and hormonal systems operate at a low level to conserve energy, to be utilised for regeneration and repair of damaged cells. Our body temperature decreases as our metabolism slows down, our heart rate and breathing maintain an optimal state. Sleep induces the repair job by rebalancing our hormonal system, strengthening our immune system, removing the damaged and dead tissue and replenishing them with new ones.

During Sleep, the level of happy hormone 'serotonin' level falls to a low level, freeing the receptors, so that those receptors can get re sensitized next morning when we get up. This is the secret of our refreshing mind in the morning and the reason, sleep deprivation causing irritation. An irritable mind has a negative impact on our moral judgments, as it impairs person's ability to integrate emotions with logic.

We need 8 hours of sleep to rejuvenate the body. When we are in stress, it breaks the normal circadian rhythm. Stress by itself does not keep us awake, but worrying about the stressors keeps us awake. Consequently, the Sleep deprivation keeps the cortisol level high and a vicious cycle sets in. The consequences of poor sleep range from total exhaustion to major health problems. Our body becomes inefficient at producing energy due to malfunctioning of our mitochondria, the powerhouse of the body. Multiple studies all over the world have proved that lack of sleep increases the risk of heart diseases, obesity, immune dysfunction and breast cancer etc.

Aging process normally affects our sleeping pattern. In our forties, level of stress hormone is elevated for most people. As the level never reaches to a low level, sleep deprivation is a common problem for this group of people. Managing stress during the daytime can reverse the pattern to some extent.

Losing weight, avoiding alcohol, caffeine before bed, performing relaxation exercises before bed, meditation, use of a good pillow and mattress, regular exercise help us in inducing a good night sleep of 8 hours.

S – Simplification of Things

Simplification of life means understanding the difference between the need and the greed. Focusing on the essential objectives of our life and letting go of the less important ones does the magic. Simplification reduces the burden we are carrying on our back throughout our life and make us stress free. The backbone of living healthy is a peaceful mind with a great concentration on improving on a daily basis in our mind, body and spirit.

We can simplify our goals into S.M.A.R.T. goals.

- S for specific,
- M for measurable,
- A for acceptable,
- R for realistic,
- T for time bound.

It is easy to accomplish a small goal and each time we finish one, we have small release of the chemical serotonin and we are ready for the next one.

'Richard Koch' in his book "Living the 80/20 way" has mentioned about the 80/20 principle. This says in simple words that 80 percent of results come from only 20 percent of cause or effect. He clearly demonstrated that 20 percent of the work we do, gives our 80% results. Therefore, instead of working hard on the rest of 80 percent of things, if we give most of our emphasis on 20 percent of the things, than the stress will be less and we achieve our goal easily.

Slowing down the pace of our work, gives us a space to take a deep breath and take rest. This will increase our productivity and health span.

Refusing for a task we are not interested to perform by saying 'No' simplifies our life in a long run.

Brain Tracy, famous business coach and author has advised, "Eat the biggest frog first". What he meant by this statement is to do the most important 20 percent of the high values jobs first. This will provide 80 percent of our achievements. The rule is to resist the temptation to clear up small things first.

Learning to manage time by scheduling based on our priority makes life simple and enjoyable. We have all the power to meet people whom we give importance and doing things, which excite us. This makes the difference.

Chapter VIII

Care for Your Aging

"It is a shame for a man to grow old without ever seeing the strength and beauty of which his body is capable".

Socrates

Aging, is an ongoing process on which we do not have a control over, but how well we will age, it depends on us. We certainly have a great role to play for delaying it for some time. We all progress at a snail's pace of 1 percent per year after the age of 30. If we carefully analyse the above hypothesis, a surprise conclusion can be reached i.e. we still have 99 percent of our body's energy and intelligence of which we are composed of, remain untouched by the aging process. Now the question arises, can we deal with these body's abilities to remain younger for a longer time?

To understand this aging phenomenon, we have to understand the two most basic biological processes undergoing in our body at any given point of time.

1. Entropy
2. Homeostasis

Entropy means the self-inflicted damage on our body, by the factors residing in our body. Every moment of our life, radioactivity, ultraviolet light, chemical toxins, pollution, random mutation, and x-ray and even by the body's own metabolism, damage our cells. Highly reactive oxygen atoms are released when food is metabolized in the cells and get bonded to many other molecules and damage their DNA.

HOMEOSTASIS is just the opposite of Entropy. It is the body's ability to normalize, replace, and correct the damage done by Entropy.

Our body is a wonderful machine. It does not respond to entropy as the old iron object rusts, though the process is same. Our body's ability to reverse and regenerate the damaging process makes us different and gives us a hope to remain younger for a longer time.

Therefore, our aim now should be to keep a balance between Entropy and Homeostasis. When the balance tips towards Entropy, we age faster and the reverse of it keeps us healthier and younger.

Our psychology play a greater role in our aging process as we no more think body and mind are separate. Someone has rightly said, "We age, faster because we see other people aging and suffering". In our subconscious mind, it is already imprinted from our childhood that we all have to pass through this with a great suffering. It is our perception, our belief that gives a boost to our aging process. We can set our bio stat of our biological age to a particular age by just bringing it into our consciousness. The moment we do it, our body will automatically organise our physiology to that particular biological age.

In our mind we should always remain young and keep our self esteem high by doing things that keep our morale high. Stress management, simple living, cultivating contentment, better interpersonal relationship, maintaining a great loving family etc are few points, on which we should work sincerely to keep ourselves young and healthy.

In this era of epigenetic, it has been proved that our environment is the key to our biological changes in our body. DNA no more controls us but our environment, controls and dictates DNA to manifest the changes in our body. This indirectly says if we give our body a favourable environment, then we can keep our self, young and disease free.

Our Biological age signifies how old our body is in terms of critical life signs and cellular processes. This is where we have a great control over our age. The biological changes are physical manifestation of our body's derangements, where reversal is possible. Few of the **markers of aging,** on which can be work, are as follows:

1. **Lean body mass**: This is the ratio of our fat mass with the fat free mass (muscle, bone, tendon, joint, ligaments). We lose on an average of 3 to 3.5 kg of muscle mass with each decade after the age of 30. The rate of loss increases after age 45. The muscle is more important for the body's overall vitality and considered as the furnace of the body metabolisms.

2. **Strength**: Aging leads to decrease in the strength of muscle due to loss of muscle bundles and motor units. This the main cause of a weaker old age.

3. **BMR**: Body's Metabolisms decrease by 2 percent per decade after the age of 20. This can be simply be reversed by leading active life.

4. **Body fat:**   The body's fat percent goes on increasing after the age of 25 years. By the time, we reach 65 it is just double the Lean body mass.

5. **Bone density:** Calcium tends to be lost from bone with age.

6. **Aerobic capacity:** by age 65, the body's ability to use oxygen efficiently decreases by 30 to 40 percent.

Researchers at TUFT University have done a major study on human aging with the above parameters of biological aging. They conclusively proved that all the above parameters are reversible to some extent with proper trainings. They concentrated on full-scale exercise program for people above 45 years. By the end of the study, they found the older man could lift heavier weight, than 25 years old could do.

The MANTRA to defeat Entropy is to regular strength exercises to build muscles. It increases the muscle tone and strengthens tendons, bones, joints and ligaments.

It increases the insulin sensitivity of cells to prevent diabetes in old age. It stops bone resorption and prevent osteoporosis in old age.

According to Deepak Chopra, exercises has to be balanced by the following 4 things

1. To do, exercise with Moderation and with gradual increasing stimulation.

2. We have to maintain the regularity.

3. Proper rest in between to allow time for repair and rejuvenate the muscle mass.

4. Active lifestyle is necessary. It is said that a minimum of 10000 steps /day to keep ourselves active.

The other important factors of healthy aging are.

1. Restful sleep,

2. Nutrition,

Experiencing *deep rest in body and mind is one of the most important steps toward* growing younger and live longer. An agitated body and mind generates entropy, decay and faster aging. Giving rest for a certain period of time, to body and mind, opens up ways to repair, create, and renew the body. Minimum six to eight hours of sleep requires for a healthy body and mind. On awakening, you should feel energetic, alert and vibrant.

Lastly, the most important factors to keep the body younger are the food we eat. The nutrients we eat built us or ruin us.Therefore,it is very important to choose our food carefully. We need a proper balanced diet for the body. It consists of plant based diet, avoiding inflammatory foods like fast food, meat, fried items etc. Fresh vegetables provide live enzymes and essential minerals, which keeps our body young. A balanced diet consists of a proper proportion of carbohydrates, fats, proteins, vitamins, minerals and water to nourish our body.

Chapter IX

Care for Your Bones and Muscles

*"How long you are going to be healthy will depend on,
how much time you are spending with yourself every day, how regularly and
How sincerely you are doing it".*

Author

I remember Mr. K P, a patient; I did a hernia operation 10 years back, when he was in his early 50 s. I remember him until now as he was one of my most active and talkative patient I ever had. He was working with a steel company as an executive. He was strong and healthy. His postoperative recovery was excellent and wound healed in time. Somehow, after one follow up, l did not have any news from him. Few months back, while crossing the out patients corridor, a very weak and frail person approached me and wished me. When he introduced himself, I was surprised to see Mr. K P in that condition. By that time, he was underweight, hypertensive, a diabetic on insulin and with severe arthritis with restricted knee joint movement. He was only 62 years old. Then he explained to me about his condition, which started deteriorating after his retirement. I could very well see how, an unplanned retirement, sedentary lifestyle, a life without a vision and lack of self-love has made the person to sufferer. There are millions of people like Mr. K P, to whom I want to send a message, so that they can prevent themselves from falling into the disease trap.

The basic framework of our body is made up of bones and muscles known as musculoskeletal system. This organ system is responsible for the movement of our body, provides the support and stability. In "care for your bones and muscles" and muscles, we are interested to create an awareness to keep this system healthy till we die, as no one wants to be bedridden before death. Unfortunately, majority of people suffer as they grow old, and become crippled due to weak bones, joints and muscles. We have to plan beforehand, for an active and pain free old age. As we have already discussed in the ageing chapter that the process of decaying starts as early as late third decades. If we take proper action and follow the rules, we can slow down the process and stay healthy and strong till we die.

Body Composition

Our muscles, bones, joints and tendons form a single unit for discussion and a major part of our lean body mass. Our bodymass in general is divided into two components. Lean body mass and fat mass. When we subtract the fat mass from the total body mass, we get the lean body mass. When we are young our lean body mass is about 55 to 96 percent of total body weight and fat mass is about 4 to 45 percent of Total body weight (TBW). The composition starts changing with age. The ratio starts reversing as our age progresses from middle age to old age.

For an average healthy male, the fat percent should be 14 to 17 percent and female should 21 to 24 percent. As we go on losing our lean body mass, mostly the muscle and bone mass, we become more and more susceptible to injury and other lifestyle diseases.

Normal Body Composition

A. Total body weight (mass) [TBW] 100%

B. Two components model:

Fat free weight (FFW) = 55–96% of TBW

Fat mass = 4–45% of TBW.

C. Tissue Components of FFW:

Muscle = 48%

Bone = 16%

Skin = 14%

Blood = 9%

Organs = 13%

Components of Fat: storage + essential fat

D. Chemical components of FFW:

Water = 72–74%

Protein = 19–21%

Bone minerals = 7%

We can assess the body composition by mainly two methods.

Body Mass Index (BMI)

This is an indirect measure of body composition and is a ratio of body weight in kilograms to height in meter square. It indicates the risks associated with high fat percentage. Higher we are in the BMI scale, higher is the mortality rate.

$$BMI = WT \text{ (weight)}/HT^2 \text{ (height in meter)}.$$

For example if my weight is 70 kg and my height is 1.67 meter, them my BMI is $70/(1.67)^2 = 25$

* Acceptable BMI	19–24 (female)	20–25 (male)
* Moderately high BMI	25–30	26–30
* Very high BMI	30+	30+

Waist Circumference

This is an indicator of health risk associated with excess fat around the waist.

Regardless of the our weight and height, waist measurement of >94 centimetres (37 inches) for man and more than 80 centimetres (31.5 inches) in female is an indicator for increased fat mass.

The aim of **"Care for your bone and muscles"** is to create awareness among the readers to work for preserving the strength of our bones, joints, tendons and muscles to keep our lean body mass stronger and healthier until we die.

Bones Care

Our skeletal system includes the bones and cartilages that provide the framework for our muscles and organs. Long bones also provide a site for our blood cell formation and have a role in immune cell formations. It is the storehouse for calcium and phosphate. Calcium is in demand for many important functions of our body. During the need, bone resorption occurs to maintain blood calcium level. Healthy bones and joints are needed to prevent injuries, sufferings from joint pain and health problems like osteoporosis.

Our bone cells are dynamic and constantly changing and in adults, it recycles 5 to 7 percent of our bone every week. We have a new skeletal system in approximately 3 to 4 months. Our bone remodelling occurs through mainly two processes. ***Continuous breakdown process is termed as bone resorption and formation is termed as deposition.*** Bone mass and shape depends on the stress placed on them or the use of it. Use it or lose it formula fits into bone remodelling. According to Wolff's law, bone forms in areas of stress and resorbed in the area of non-stress. Remodelling of bones for strength and mass gets influenced by the physical activity of the individual.

Only 1 gm of calcium present in our extracellular fluid as compared to 1150 gm of calcium in bone tissue. About 4% of the body weight comes from mineral weight. Therefore, if we weigh 50 kg by the age 25 then, the approximately 2 kg of minerals will be there in our body. As our age progresses, at the age 50 and if we weigh 75 then, the mineral weigh should be 3 kg, but unfortunately most of the time we are in negative balance, i.e. about 2 kg or less. The bone calcium and phosphate salts are responsible for the hardness of the bone matrix. The BMD (Bone Mineral Density) determined our bone health. When our blood calcium level falls, body tries to compensate it by bone resorption (breakdown).

Ninety-five percent of peak bone mass is achieved by the age 20 and in mid 30 s; it reaches to its 100 percent. It gets influenced by, mechanical factors, age, nutrition, hormonal level and genetics. For a healthy bone, we have to maintain this peak bone mass by paying careful attention to modifiable factors like nutritional status, hormonal status and activity level.

Physical activity increase the mechanical forces on bones, which stimulate the physiological changes in bone cells that allow bones to be modelled and remodelled. Our bones are adapted to the challenges put on it in the form of magnitude, rate and the distribution of load on the bone.

Recommended activity for Bone Health:

1. Weight bearing physical activity induces new bone formation and strengthening of bone. Brisk walking, jogging, running, climbing stairs, jumping rope, dancing, weight lifting, Hath yoga, football are few examples. In older man and women who performed strength training, has increased bone mineral density, bone size and strength. At least 30 minutes of training daily is recommended.

2. Eat green vegetables as it contains many micronutrients, vitamins needed during bone formation and protects bones from getting demineralised in young women.

3. A balanced diet with proper protein supplements helps protect bone health in old age.

4. Calcium supplements through eating food containing high calcium is recommended, Spinach, beets, tomatoes, sweet potatoes, cabbage, broccoli, juices fortified with calcium are bone health friendly foods.

5. Enough exposure to sun for vitamin D is necessary with food rich in Vitamin D like, fish, cheese etc. This helps in absorption of calcium from the food.

6. Vitamin K2 plays an important role in bone metabolism and it can prevent osteoporosis and fracture.

7. Recent research has found that olive oil; soybeans, blueberries and food rich in omega 3, like fish oil and flaxseed oil also have bone boosting capacity.

8. We have to cut down high salt coating food as high sodium causes body to lose calcium and induces osteoporosis.

9. We should avoid addicting agents like alcohol, coffee, tea, and soft drinks, which decreases calcium absorption.

Osteoporosis and Bone Health

Osteoporosis means "porous bones", which leads to compromised bone strengthen and risk of fracture of bones. Osteoporosis is becoming one of the most common health problems all over the world due to adaptation of unhealthy and sedentary lifestyle. This results from an imbalance between bone formation and bone resorption. After the age 30, bone mass stops increasing and bone, resorption starts because of sedentary lifestyle.

The following are few of the risk factors associated with osteoporosis.

1. Genetic: race, sex, family history

2. Nutritional: excessive alcohol intake, low calcium intake, high protein intake

3. Lifestyle: lack of physical activity, smoking

4. Physiological: Delayed menarche, amenorrhea, and early menopause

Nutrition for Osteoporosis

The main components of bone formation are calcium, magnesium, potassium, Vitamins D, E, K2, beta-carotene, and proteins. When our body gets all these things from food we eat, we have healthy bones. Calcium gets absorbed in the intestine when the calcium to phosphorus ratio in the food is 2:1.

1. Fresh vegetables

2. Nuts

3. Ragi

4. Dates

5. Fruits

6. Pulses and legumes

7. Egg

8. Omega 3 fatty acids (Flaxseeds or pumpkin seeds, fish)

9. Calcium fortified foods

"Care for your bones," recommends building bone through high impact activities up to third decades. From middle age, we have to maintain it by reducing bone loss and preventing falls. This can be achieved by emphasizing on activities, which challenge the postural system and resistance training for loading muscles and bones. The principle of reversibility is also true. The benefit of exercise is lost when we ceases exercising. We have to do it daily, and with consistently.

Muscle and Tendon Care

Our body has more than 400 muscles, which accounts for 40 to 45% of the adult male body weight and 23 to 25 percent of adult female body weight. This is the largest metabolically active organ of our body and considered as the 'Blast Furnace' of the human metabolic system. Muscle contractions provide the basis of all human movement. Tendons are strong bands of tissue that attaches muscles to bone and transfers the force across the joints. The more active and healthy our muscle mass is, the more fit we are. There are three types of muscles in our body.

1. Skeletal,

2. Smooth

3. Cardiac

Out of three, we can control skeletal muscles voluntarily and rest of the two is involuntary. We can be increase skeletal muscles strength voluntarily by working on them. However, when we do workout for skeletal muscles, we also increase the strength and vascularity of our cardiac and intestinal smooth muscles. Taking care of muscle mass, indirectly takes care of the all other systems. Muscles cells also act as an endocrine organ as it has a role in the glucose metabolism if properly trained. *In type II diabetes, where the issue is insulin insensitivity, it activates and relocates the GLUT 4, insulin dependent receptor pathway and utilises the excess glucose and controls diabetic.*

There is only one way, by which we can take care of our muscle mass. *By doing regular workouts with proper muscles training principles we can build up our muscle mass and improve our cardiac, respiratory, gastrointestinal, immune functions of our body.* Tendons are prone for injury due to inappropriate movement of body and joints. Avoiding unnatural movements and giving proper rest to injured tendon can prevent further damage and increase the scope of repair. Proper warm up and gradually building the intensity level can prevent the injury.

Muscles Training (Strength Training)

Muscular fitness can be obtained through mainly Resistance training programs. Resistance training is a systematic program of exercises involving the exertion of force against a load with a goal of developing strength, endurance, and hypertrophy of muscle system (Devies and Barnes, 72). It is commonly known as weight training.

"Care for your health," recommends resistance training for healthy children, adolescents, adults and older adults. Resistance training should be done under proper supervision, breathing control and with appropriate load.

Warming up the body is the prerequisite to start a strength training session. It raises our body temperature and increases the circulation. We can prevent injury and soreness of muscle by doing a proper warm up. The simplest thing to do is to lift lighter weights for few minutes before you go for a load of your normal training session.

Specificity is the first principle. It should be very much specific to the individual's goal like muscular fitness, athletic performance enhancement or body building competitions.

Four things are to be looked for muscular fitness

1. Muscle strength,
2. Hypertrophy (increase in size),
3. Power
4. Endurance

Overload: In resistance, training requires proper load selection, volume, and frequency and rest interval. Most of the complications of strength training occur due to improper load during exercise. We have to choose our load correctly and progressively. The work done per session (volume) of resistance training should be, carefully increased in due course of time.

The frequency of exercise session has to be, planned according to the need. Health related fitness requires at least 2 sessions of strength training per week and the more we do, the more benefit we get from the same training, in due course of time.

The most important of overload is the rest period in between two sessions for the **recovery** of the injured muscles. Proper rest and adequate diet gradually lead to adaptation of the muscle to that particular load and prevents injury and soreness of that muscle group. Ideally 24 to 48 hours of rest is needed to load the same muscle groups for the next session.

Progression of the load or stimulus is necessary once our body gets adapted to a particular weight. This is the basis of progressive resistance exercise. We can achieve progression by increasing the load, the repetitions, and the number of sets or the frequency of workout.

Maintenance is the final principle of strength training. Once the required strength or endurance has been achieved, it is important to maintain it by reduced frequency of sessions.

Pre and post workout food is as important as the workout. Proper maintenance of hydration is very important. So keeping a bottle of water during workout is essential. It is wise to take a low GI (Glycemic index) food, 20 to 30 minutes before workout. Fruits like banana and apple are the right kind for the purpose. We need proteins for the repair of the injured muscle cells. So diet rich in proteins are needed. Whey proteins are a good source of essential amino acids and are recommended by many. Vitamins and mineral with antioxidants helps in the recovery by neutralising the free radicals generated during exercise.

Care for Your Joints and Ligaments

Joints are the point where two bones connect with each other with the help of ligaments and provide movement according to the need of the structure.

Restriction of joint moment due to lack of proper care and misuse has become an epidemic throughout the world and millions of people are suffering from severe pain and getting crippled. If due care and precautions are taken by the time we reach middle age, these suffering can be prevented.

"Care for your health," recommends the following precautions for joint health.

Regular joint movements in the form of exercise should be a routine for every person irrespective of sex. As we are now living a sedentary lifestyle, our joints are getting stiffer due to less movement. So be active and move your joints whenever you get an opportunity. Movement should be in all the direction, a joint naturally has.

Strengthening the muscles and tendons holding the joints can increase the support of the joint and reduces the direct stress on it. Strength training to increase the strength and power of our spinal and paraspinal muscles, which supports our spine, can prevent backache and disc prolapse. This is the reason the porters who carry huge loads on head, hardly suffers from backbone problems. Training to strengthen the hip, thigh and leg muscles prevent hip and knee joint pain to a great extent. Strength training also strengthens the corresponding bones resulting in a strong and healthy joint. We should take all the precautions, not to over strain the joints by taking proper rest.

Maintaining a proper weight can be a boon to our joints. We suffer when our joints cannot bear our bodyweight and the joint space reduces due to compression. Reduce space lead to more friction and increased inflammation oedema of joint space. This causes restriction of movement, pain and suffering.

Yoga for Muscle and Joint Care

Yoga Asana have often considered as a form of good exercises for joints. They are techniques, which place the body in position that cultivate awareness, relaxation, concentration and meditation. SukshmaVyayama (Fine Exercises) is concerned with releasing tension from the joints. These are excellent for 'joint care', as regular practice brings awareness and coordination between bones, joints, ligaments, muscles etc. These are minor exercise from toes to head.

Position/Posture

While doing all the joints movements we should sit straight having the angle of 90 degree between our legs and upper portion of your body. Keeping hands on either sides of our back let us join our legs. Our back, neck and head should be straight.

Relaxation

While doing joints movements, if we feel tired, we must relax for few seconds.

Relaxation in the Sitting Posture

Let us Make little gap between our legs. Let us lie our feet flat, bending our back little backward and tilting our neck in any one direction. Let us feel relaxed and do normal abdominal breathing.

Leg Joints Movements

Base position- Let us sit with the leg outstretched, feet close together but not touching. Back, neck, head should be straight, 90 degree to thighs.

1. **Toe bending** – Let us move toes backwards and forward 10 times. Inhalation as the toes goes backwards and exhalation as the toe goes forward.

2. **Ankle bending** – Let us move feet forward and backward from the ankle joint for 10 times. Inhale as the feet move backward; Exhale as the feet move forward.

3. **Ankle rotation** – keeping the leg shoulder width we should rotate our feet in both clockwise and anticlockwise direction for five times. With the practice, we can gradually increase rotations until 10 times. Next, rotate both the feet together in the same direction, clock and anti-clockwise direction 10 times each. Thirdly, let us rotate both the feet from the ankle

joint but in opposite directions, 10 times each. We should do Inhalation during upward movement and exhalation on downward movement.

4. **Leg movements** – let us keep our left leg over right knee such that our left foot should remain completely out. Then rotate left foot in both clockwise and anticlockwise direction for five times. While rotation, we can hold left toe with our right hand and put left hand on the left ankle. Now let us lift left leg until it reaches our right thigh. Putting the left hand on the left knee and moving it up and down for 10 times. After moving it up and down, in the same position let us rotate our left leg in both clockwise and anticlockwise direction for 5 times. Again lifting the left leg let, we try to touch heel to our navel. We should repeat all these steps with our right leg as well.

5. Let us join our legs. Contract and relax our knees for 20 times.

6. **Butterfly flapping** – let us join the bottoms of our feet, cross our fingers and put them below the feet. Let us bring our feet closer to us as far as possible and flip our legs up and down for 10 times. Initially we may feel pain in our thigh muscles.

7. **Body bending** – Let us take our legs apart from each other as far as possible. Lift our hands on either side. Let us turn to our left and try to touch the left toes with our right hand. See towards left. Similarly turn to our right and try to touch the right toes with our left hand. See towards right. Do it for 10 times.

Chapter X

Care for Your Food and Fluid

"We all live a borrowed life. The air we inhale and the food we eat is a gift from the plant kingdom. The microorganisms residing in our body provide half of the genetic instructions of our survival. It's a paradox that in our everyday living we ignore them, underestimate them and destroy them".

Author

"Let food be thy medicine and medicines be thou food". 2000 years ago Hippocrates, the father of medicine has given emphasis on food through his teachings.

Foods we eat are one of the essential commodities of life, without which we cannot survive for a long time. It is the fuel for our body. It provides raw materials to our cellular factory, which produces required products to operate, maintain and repair our body parts. We get the energy to maintain this body, from the food we eat and the oxygen we inhale. Each one of us is genetically programmed to unlock the energy of the sun that is stored in the naturally occurring food material like plants and seeds, present in our immediate environment. Our body finds it difficulties to process food full of chemical preservatives and colouring agents.

The nutrients in food are nothing but molecular messengers that guides our cells to perform either constructively for a better health or negatively towards illness. So in a way food can serve as one of the best preventive agent for us. If we can identify individually, the food, which are draining our energy every day and recognize the food, which enhances our energy, the confusion of food,can be solved forever. For a healthy life, we need to consume food, which will cause minimal damage and maximal repair of our cells. Recent advancement in nutritional science has identified many of the factors responsible for our good health and proved that food as the culprit for our illness.

The basic understanding of the energy in food looks simple but it is not so. We get our energy from the three major macromolecules carbohydrate, fats and proteins. However, the new research gives equal importance to the micronutrients like, minerals, vitamins, enzymes and amino acids for the generations of energy in our body. Therefore, the food containing only macronutrients and deficient of micronutrients will not serve the purpose and in fact cause damage by utilizing the stored micronutrients present in our body.

When food passes through our digestive system, it gets broken down into glucose, fatty acids, amino acids, vitamins, minerals, water etc and gets absorbed into the circulation. Once in the circulation, it reaches our energy factory Mitochondria and with the help of oxygen we inhale, produces the energy needed for the functioning of the body. Energy formed is stored in our body in the form of a molecule known as ATP and available for our use. It is known as universal energy currency of the body. Once the energy is released for use, it goes back to cell and is converted to the parent molecule ADP. Now it is ready again to get charged to become ATP, like a microscopic recyclable battery. Our body creates trillions of ATP every moment and each one get recycled thousands of times. Our mitochondria can capture only about 40% of energy stored in our food, in an ideal, stress free and unpolluted environment.

Studies conducted by Harvard school of public health, it has been found that most of the adult population are deficient in vitamins and minerals because of the changed food habits. The metabolic processes in our body have to continue throughout our lifetimes for our survival. *When there is a scarcity of micronutrients in our food, our body gets its required vitamins and minerals from the tissues and nearby cells. This type of sharing makes the donor cells or tissue weak and diseased, in due course of time.*

The food we eat are nothing but a collection of genetic signalling molecules. For example, if we eat sugar, then the sugar molecules signals our DNA to produce insulin. If we drink tea or coffee, it signals our DNA to activate our nervous system to alert our mind.

The food we eat supply materials needed to build our body through a process known as anabolism.

Carbohydrates are the main energy supplier to the body. 60% of our energy comes from carbohydrates. Two terminologies in carbohydrates metabolism are very important and we should have clear understanding of them.

Glycemic Index (GI)

Glycemic Load (GL).

Glycemic index is how quickly sugar is absorbed from the food into circulation. A high Glycemic index food raises the sugar level immediately due to quick absorption and there after an abrupt fall when the glucose get utilised.

Glycemic load is a measure of the amount of a food actually delivered to the cells. It measures both the quantity and quality of carbohydrates. GL is calculated as follows;

$$GL = (GI \times Carbohydrate\ (g)\ content\ per\ portion)/100$$

For example, an apple contains 13 gms of carbohydrates and GI of 38

$$GL = 38 \times 13/100 = 5$$

Similarly a potato contain 14 gms of carbohydrate, but has GI 86,

$$GL = 86 \times 14/100 = 12$$

Low GL food is good as it prevents glycation due to slow and small glucose delivery.

Proteins are our building blocks. Proteins are used for many of the important cell functions like muscle building to formation of enzymes, hormones, neurotransmitters etc.

Fats are required to maintain the integrity of the cell wall and supply energy to the body in emergency.

The Food we eat also causes a lot of damage to our body during their normal metabolic events. The following three processes are mainly responsible for the damages that occur in our body.

1. Oxidation
2. Inflammation
3. Glycation

Oxidation

During the metabolism of our food, many highly destructive molecules called free radical are produced in our cells. Free radicals are the molecules that have unpaired electrons. These free radicals are always looking to make bond with other molecules by giving electron or take away electrons from them and this process is known as oxidation. Because of this type of electron transfer, these free radicals have the capacity to damage our DNA and other cell structures. This happens when our food contain more free radical producing food like, meat, refined sugar, trans fats, fried items etc. Stress, air pollution, poor breathing technique, radiation, drugs, aging processes and infections increase the oxidation process.

We have an inbuilt mechanism to counter these damaging substances. Problem arises when theses evil substances out numbers our neutralizing materials. Increasing the intake of food containing antioxidants like berries, citrus fruits, green leafy vegetables, carrots, tomatoes and green tea etc, help to neutralize these damaging substances.

"Care for your health," recommends at least five servings of fruits and vegetables every day and plenty of water. Fruits and vegetables comes with a natural supply of minerals like, calcium, magnesium, phosphorus, iron and vitamins like Beta carotene, Vitamin C, Vitamin B complex.

Inflammation

Inflammation, is the body's defence against foreign invaders to our body, it is a natural process. Inflammation is a reaction in our cells causing redness, swelling, heat, and pain. We can call it our immune reaction to save us from outer attack. Certain food we ingest can introduce pro inflammatory substances into our body and can produce cytokines, which sets inflammation, and damage our body. Nearly everything natural and fresh is anti-inflammatory. Everything artificial promote inflammation, especially refined sugar, starches, milk products and trans fats.

Some foods are neither inflammatory or anti inflammatory, like grains fall into the category of neutral. However, few react to Gluten containing grains and produce inflammatory reaction in the body. Some of the vegetables like tomato, potato, hot peppers contain inflammatory substance called solanine. Some are intolerant to this chemical. We should eliminate the food we are intolerant to from our diet.

Genetically we all are different with different metabolic capabilities. Geographically, depending on the local food availability our body is tuned to digest and accommodate certain foods. *So it will be improper to advice same food profile to all.* Food should be very much personalised according to the need. We should out rightly reject the food, which brings uneasiness when taken. We will be able to do this when we will listen to our body and carefully plan for ourselves.

ANTI INFLAMMATORY	INFLAMMATORY
Fresh, Unprocessed	Old, Rancid, Processed, Micro waved, Skimmed, Canned, adulterated
Fruits	meats and poultry
Vegetables	potato, Tomatoes, hot peppers
Herbs	drugs and medicine
Water, Herbal Tea	soft drink, milk, juices
plant oils like Olive, nuts oil,	Animal fats, Commercial Oils, Corn oil, palm oil
Food cooked at low flame	Fried, Baked, grilled, broiled at high temperature
soya foods	Dairy Products
Nuts and dried fruits	Candies, chocolate bars
Natural sweet fruits	Sugar, artificial sweeteners
Water	dehydration

Glycation

When our body has excess of sugar molecules, it is bound to the proteins of our body through a process called glycation. As we are nothing but a protein machine, our cellular structures gets transformed and the normal functioning of our body gets affected. We age faster, and our hormonal, enzymatic functions are deranged due to alterations of the proteins structures. The more quickly sugar floods our circulation, the more damage it does to our body's structures and functions through glycation. Avoiding processed foods, sugary drinks, ice creams and candies, energy bars, can stop the glycation process and save us from early damage.

Complex carbohydrates like oatmeal, Whole meal rye, all bran cereal, muesli, lentils, beans, apple, cherry, grapefruit, tomato, oranges, kiwi are foods which causes least glycation because of slow release and high Glycemic load (GL).

Eating food rich in water is one of the most important advices, whichcan be given to anyone interested to lead a healthy lifestyle. Water consists of 70 percent of our body and it is the best solvent in existence until date. Water acts as a carrier of the toxic by products of our metabolism, to the different excretory organs, like kidneys, skin, lungs to remove them from our body. Fruits vegetables, sprouts are the food rich with water and act as cleansing agent. It is advisable to keep 70 percent of our diet rich in water containing food.

"Care for your food" advocate, salad with every meal, sprouts in morning and fruits in empty stomach and in between meals.

We should know little about the way we combine food when we eat. The carbohydrates, proteins and fats we eat are digested in our body at a different speed and different medium. All three require different enzymes and digestive solutions for digestion. When we eat foods having opposite digestive requirements in the same sitting, then it is considered as bad food combinations. This results in abdominal bloating, cramps etc. For example, proteins require an acidic environment and pepsin, while carbohydrates required an alkaline environment and ptyalin. When taken together, acid and alkaline solution neutralizes each other, resulting in slow and poor digestion. This is the reason we feel tired and sluggish after returning from a grand party. Undigested food materials become a source for putrefaction and fermentation, leading to allergy and infection. Few important things to remember about food combinations are

1. Carbohydrates and animal proteins should not be taken together.
2. Fruits should be taken alone in empty stomach.
3. Grains should be taken separately from proteins.
4. The rule is first protein than carbohydrates.
5. Five hour pause is necessary before the next big meal to reboot the digestive juice secretions and start the next cycle of digestion.
6. No proteins or fat (meat, fish, poultry, eggs) with refined and concentrated sugar (commercial fruit juice, sauces, pastry, soft drink, candy).
7. Proper chewing is necessary to mix starch foods with ptyalin secreted from salivary gland and digest it, as ptyalin does not act in acid medium.
8. Do not drink sweetened drink and eat breads at the same time as Sweets inhibit secretions of ptyalin.
9. Select your protein wisely and select any one of the proteins at a time with each meal in order to avoid superfluous amino acids.
10. Drink water at least 20 to 30 minutes after a meal. This reduces the dilution of digestive juices in stomach.
11. Eat regularly; maintain timetable; do not skip meals.

12. Never, eat whenever you are in hurry. Eat in leisure, attentively and with gratitude.

13. Eat in moderation. There is a saying for eating, "stop before you are stuffed". Stop eating the moment you feel full, that is when you are 80% full.

14. Plan your meals around available vegetarian foods and add fish and poultry in between. Do not get upset when you break the rules. Instead, enjoy it.

Eternal Rules of Eating

1. Always enjoy eating, rather than just gulping.
2. Never be in a hurry to eat. Relaxed and take you own time.

Vitamins Facts

Vitamins are natural substances, needed for our vital growth but are not manufactured in our body. We get these molecules from the food we ingest on a day to day basis. Vitamins are either fat soluble or water soluble. We have 13 vitamins present in our food. We must obtain vitamins from natural foods or dietary supplements in order to sustain life. Vitamins are an integral part of our enzyme system, responsible for the thousands of chemical reactions occurring inside our body. Processed foods are deficient of vitamins.

Water soluble vitamins are the B group (B1, B2, B3, B5, B6, B12 and folate, biotin) and C. These water soluble vitamins cannot be stored in our body, so we need to take them daily. The best sources of vitamin B complex are as follows.

1. Whole meal bread, brown rice, poultry, eggs, fish and meat.
2. Legumes, fresh vegetables, bananas, cheese etc.

Vitamin C is a potent antioxidant. It is present abundantly in all citrus fruits like, lemon, oranges, and sprouts, tomatoes, broccoli, papayas, cherries, green chillies, Guavas, Fat-soluble Vitamins arre A, D, E, and K. Theses vitamins can be stored in our body. The main storage organ for fat soluble vitamins is liver. The best parts of fat-soluble vitamins are that their potency remains intact after cooking also.

Vitamin A is available in food of animal origin like fish, eggs and meat. Some food of plant origin having beta-carotene, available in fruits and vegetables like Carrots, dark green leafy vegetables, pumpkins and apricots are good source beta carotene.

Vitamin D is plays an important role in body's use in calcium and phosphorus. Primary source of vitamin D is oily fish like salmon and cod liver oil. Sunlight is an important source of vitamin D.

Vitamin E is a wonderful antioxidant. About 60% of vitamin D comes from vegetables oil, fruits, grains, nuts, etc.

Vitamin K is naturally produced by our microbiota. Good source of this vitamin K includes spinach, cabbage, cauliflower, and oils like soybean oil and olive oil.

Fruits Facts

We are biologically adapted to eat fruits. Dr. Alan walker an anthropologist, in his research on fossil teeth, found that our ancestors were predominantly fruit eaters. Fruits have the highest water content of any food. Because of the high water content and abundance of vitamins, minerals, amino acids and carbohydrates, it helps our body to cleanse the build up residue from the system. Fruits are the perfect nutrients or our cellular health. Fruits contain all the five essentials of life, which are glucose, amino acids, minerals, fatty acids, and vitamins. The proportion of these life elements are as follows;

Glucose- 90%

Amino acids- 4% to 5%

Minerals- 3% to 4%

Fatty acids- 1+%

Vitamins- 1+%

The only advice for fruits consumption is to eat **FRESH**. Fruits lose its all life giving elements if we alter it by any means. The Golden rule is no cooking, no mixing with other macronutrients and even juicing of fruits.

The other important instruction for fruit consumption is to eat it in empty stomach. A minimum of 20 to 30 minutes gap should be given before other foods are consumed. Banana, dates and other dried food take little more time, about 45 minutes to 1 hour to leave stomach. We have to wait at least 2 hour after taking a major meal, for fruit consumption.

The electrolyte rich fruits act as a diuretic and induce urination more frequently. This leads to increase in the elimination of our nitrogenous waste and chlorides. Fruits have an alkalisation property, which promotes elimination of toxic wastes from intestine and neutralises the harmful effect of acid forming foods. High fibre contain of fruits has a good laxative effect on our body.

Thrifty Gene

These are the genes, which enables individuals to efficiently collect and process food to deposit as fat during period of food abundance in order to provide for periods of food shortage. This thrifty gene is activated, when we do dieting and restrict our food to lose weight. With an anticipation of famine in the future, it conserves the food we eat in the form of fat. This leads to weight gain and we become weak due to less food being available for maintenance of our basal metabolism.

Fasting

Fasting affects our body metabolism to a greater extent. Within first six hours of fasting, our body fuel itself from the stored liver glycogen and fatty acids of our adipose tissue. As the fasting progresses, our stored glucose gets exhausted and body fat continues to be broken down for energy purpose. As our red blood cells and nervous system needs only glucose for energy purpose, they refuse the energy generated from fatty acids for use. In that particular circumstance, our body will produce glucose from the proteins available in our lean body tissue. Therefore, as the fasting continues for more than 24 hours, the protein breakdown increases. When the fasting continues for a week or more, 90% of the energy comes from the process of glucose formation from our lean body mass. When the lean body mass declines by 50%, death occurs. It is advisable to take glucose throughout the fasting period, to prevent the loss of muscle mass. Glucose in the form of fruits and juices are recommended during fasting.

Fluid: Water

Water is our life and has remarkable potential to keep us young and healthy. It is the most abundant chemical present on our planet. We are 70 percent to

80 percent water depending on the amount of fat we have. Our fat contains little water approximately 10 percent and our plasma contains 90 percent of water. The skin, muscles and internal organs contain about 70 to 80 percent of water. Our bones consist of 22 percent water. Mother's milk, juicy fruits and succulent vegetables contain 87 percent water. Nearly 98% of our intestinal, gastric, salivary and pancreatic juices are water. Because of difference in the body composition between two sexes, female has got little lower water percentage. Two thirds of our body fluids present inside cells and one-third outside the cells but in between the cells and in our blood vessels. Cellular water equilibrium is the key to life. Cells do not function optimally when there is an imbalance in the water distribution. The volume of water in our extracellular space is responsible for maintenance of our blood pressure. It is magnetic and electrical properties are key to the cellular health. Water is responsible for the maintenance of our body temperature and maintaining the pH balance of our body. Water, act as the coolest lubricant for our joints.

The great dissolving power of water helps to dissolve variety of substances of our body into it. These soluble substances are then transported to 100 trillions of cells of our body to keep them healthy and alive.

- The fluid running in our body contains hormones, red blood cells, protective immune cells, micronutrients for the use of our cells.

- Our mucus membranes need plenty of water to keep them soft and smooth.

- Water holds our cells together by remaining inside and outside the cells to give a shape to us, just as sand holds to each other when they are wet.

- Water is necessary for every chemical and enzymatic reaction inside our body.

- Water helps in lubricating joints and cushioning inter vertebral discs.

- Water regulates body temperature.

- The toxic by-products of our cellular metabolism also get carried away through this fluid of our body as urine, perspiration, tear and breathe. We lose about 3 litres of fluid every day as insensible loss, perspiration, urine, and stool. The moment we are deprived of this wonder molecules, our cells will die due to the deficiencies of required nutrients and toxic overload. Nothing can substitute the water molecules of our body.

One of the root causes of today's ill health is the decreased water intake and overconsumption of fluids in the form of tea, coffees, alcohol and other beverages. These beverages may be able to substitute the volume but it is like an acid rain over a cornfield. These liquids have no cellular utility and act only as stimulants. Once there is excessive stimulation of nervous system due to stress or illness, we normally postpone the duty of drinking water and make our cells dehydrated and sick. Depression is one of the most common manifestations of chronic dehydration, as many of the neurotransmitter formed in the brain requires water for proper functioning. Many of the chronic medical conditions like headaches, arthritis, indigestion, chronic fatigue, constipation are linked to chronic dehydration.

Living a healthy life needs sufficient amount of right kind of liquid in the form of pure water, fresh fruits, vegetables and their juices. For a better brain health, we have to supply sufficient fluids to keep the 15 billion brain cells properly hydrated.

How Much Dehydrated Are We?

We are not aware of the hydration status of our body, most of the time and are never interested to measure how much water we are consuming every day. Approximately 80% of people are chronically dehydrated. It is very difficult to diagnose chronic dehydration, as the dehydration occurs inside the cells. Because of the great adaptive power of our body, our cells manage to function reasonably well for some time. This is the reason for which we are unable to notice the chronic dehydration for a long time. By the time we notice the damage, it is too late. If we lose water of about 2 percent of our body mass, it is considered as a significant loss and affects our performance. Colour of our urine may sometime indicate the dehydration status by its darker yellow colour, but only in severe cases. We can safely assume that we are dehydrated to some extent, unless we are taking more than half the amount of our body weight in fluid ounce per day. For example if someone weigh 180 pounds than, he should take minimum 90 fluid ounce of water per day.

Acute dehydration is symptomatic. It may be presented as dryness of mouth, headaches, muscle cramps, fatigue. This happens mostly when we do strenuous activities and lose water through sweating. This needs medical attention to replenish the volume in a short period of time. Most of us are driving our body, with the water level on the reserve mode. If we do not replenish the volume in proper time, we have to face the danger of failure of our engine (our body).

The Water is a simple molecule and present abundantly around us, so most of the time its benefits are not well appreciated by all of us. Recommended quantity is bare minimum of 64 fluid ounces (2 litres) or more of water per day. As tea, coffee induces dieresis, we lose water frequently from our body, it is recommended to add one or more glass of water for every cup of coffee we drink.

We have **three sources for water** to get into our body.

- First is the amount of water we drink,
- second from the fresh fruits and vegetables we eat
- Lastly from the metabolism of our macromolecules

Best way to rehydrate our self is to begin slowly and increase it gradually over a period of time. When we start rehydrating, very quickly the frequency of urination increases initially. However, with time, our body adapts to this increased amount of fluid, by increasing the body reserve of water.

We become dehydrated when water loss is 1% of our total water content. Drinking 500 ml of water increase the metabolic rate by 30% because of water induced thermo genesis. Water consumed before meal can reduce energy intake among non-obese individuals.

Conversation Chart

64 fluid ounce = 1.9 litres

8 fluid ounce = 250 ml

1 cup = 225 ml

1 pint us liquid = 473.17 ml

1 quart US liquid = 946.35 ml (1 litter)

1 kg = 2.20 pounds = 35.27 ounce

Drinking right kind and amount of water is our best natural protection against most of the viral and other infectious diseases.

Care for Your Health Recommendations

1. Drink minimum of eight glass of water per day. Add one glass of water for each time we drink a cup of tea or coffee.

2. To measure exact consumption of water, drink water from glass.

3. Avoid drinking beverages like, tea, coffee, soft drinks, diet cola, as these substances facilitate water loss.

4. Eat fresh fruits, bursting with life giving water.

5. Never drink from bottle as most of the time, we just take one or two gulps of water to satisfy our thirst but not our dehydration.

Chapter XI

Care for Your Protectors

"We are rewarded with a healthy body and mind, when we find the purpose of our life and work towards its fulfilment. That is the time when each and every cells of our body dances in harmony with nature, which brings health".

Author

We are born fighters. We are born with an army of protectors who take care of us, all throughout our life. Without the warrior cells we cannot survive for a minute. From the time, we are born until death our body comes across millions of adverse conditions and events, which could have eliminated us from this planet. Fortunately, God has provided us with proper instruments to fight against all odds. Nature has provided us the tools to fight. It is we, who have to learn to use it to our own advantage.

Our body comes with **natural barriers,** which provides protection from the external offenders. Someone has rightly said, "Good fences make good neighbours". Our skin is the biggest first line defence against many pathogens. Other exposed areas of our body, where there are no skin lining, our body secretion like saliva, gastrointestinal fluids, lachrymal discharges, vaginal secretions, nasal mucosal discharge etc are nature's gift to us for preventing pathogens to enter and protects us from harmful chemicals and organisms. Modern living style has totally changed our natural environment and forced us to live in highly polluted atmosphere. Our body is not tuned to face so much pollution but does its assigned job to protect us. When our protectors fail to protect us, diseases step into our life. It is our duty to keep this barrier intact for a healthy life.

We have a complete and independent system in our body to protect us from different type of invaders known as **immune system.** Immunity is defined as the ability of the body to defend itself from infections, diseases and other unwanted biological invasion. We all have to encourage our immune system to stay healthy and powerful, so that we can live a healthy life. It is our umbrella, which will save us from getting wet from the rain of many diseases. We are born with a certain degree of defence mechanism, coded in the genes of our primitive bone marrow cells known as innate immunity. These are our white blood corpuscles (WBC), macrophages that initiate inflammatory reaction to eliminate foreign invaders. In addition, we passively get mother's immunity for sometime after birth.

Different organs, like bone marrow, thymus, spleen, lymph nodes, produce immune cells of our body. Different cell types like phagocytes, which includes granulocytes, macrophages, dendritic cells and lymphocytes like T and B cells work together to activate the immune system.

When we grow, we come across many more foreign substances, bacteria, viruses and toxins, which are new to our body. These invaders force our body to build defence against them, known as acquired or **adaptive immunity**. Here the key role is played by lymphocytes and is highly specific. Vaccine induced immunity is an example of **acquired immunity**. Adaptive immunity can be active or passive depending on whetherthese are generated by the cells or actively transferred from other individual.

Our **microbiota** is the next powerful protector we have, as it is responsible for formation of 90% of our immune cells. As we have discussed earlier, our friendly microbes residing in our body outnumber our normal cells. Gut microbiome regulates our natural immune response and determines the risk of chronic illnesses. Making sure that our bacterial flora intact is important for healthy functioning of the immune system. Eating naturally fermented foods, avoiding antibacterial soap and avoiding unnecessary antibiotics can improve our microbiota and thus improves our immunity.

Antioxidants are molecules that protect us from free radicals, which cause oxidation reaction in our body, by neutralising them. Free radicals are simple molecules with one or more unpaired electrons, and are highly unstable. To become stable, the free radicals steal electrons from another molecule, making it unstable and can cause permanent damage to it. Oxygen is the life giving molecules without which we cannot survive. Energy is generated when the food we eat is oxidised by oxygen we inhale. As oxidation reaction causes rusting of iron and damage it, an unwelcome oxidation reaction can cause damage to our cells including our DNA and proteins.

Antioxidants always donate an electron to the free radicals, stabilize it and stop the chain reaction. Every moment we generate millions of free radicals but most of them get neutralized by the antioxidants produced in our body and from the food, we ingest. Unfortunately, because of our changed lifestyle and food habits, the proportion of free radicals generated is very high as compared to the antioxidants present in our body. Stress, fast food, alcohol, pollution, smoking, emotional distress, drugs, infections, injuries, radiation are few of the factors responsible for increased free radicals formation leading to lifestyle diseases including cancer, obesity, diabetes, hypertension, heart attack.

Fruits, green leafy vegetables, Garlic, Spinach, Beet, Orange, Strawberry, Cherry, Onion, Corn Plum, eggs, nuts are few which contain a very high concentration of antioxidants and help us to lead a healthy life. Tea both black and green varieties, have much higher antioxidants properties. Brewing both varieties of tea with boiling water, 84% of the antioxidant properties are activated within five minutes. Rest 13% are extracted in the next five minutes. Therefore, to reap the benefits of antioxidant properties of tea, it has to be brewed for 10 minutes.

Some of the natural antioxidants are Vitamin A present in the form of Retinoic acid, Carotenoids present in our colourful fruits and vegetables. Beta Carotene, lutein, Lycopene, Zeaxanthin, Alpha carotene and Cryptoxanthin, Vitamin C, Vitamin E, are few powerful antioxidants present in different coloured vegetables and fruits. Few minerals like selenium, zinc and hormones like melatonin are frequently being used for the treatment of chronic diseases to reduce the damage caused by oxidation reactions in our body.

"Care for your health "recognizes stress as biggest threats to our immune system. Dr. Bruce Lipton in his book 'Biology of belief' mentioned that our survival mechanism is mainly divided into two categories: growth and protection. Though we need both the mechanism for survival, they cannot operate optimally at the same time. When we are in stress, automatically we switch into the protection mode and our sympathetic nervous system (SNS) prepares our body for vigorous activities. Our body releases stress hormones like, epinephrine, nor epinephrine and cortisol and prepares itself for a fight- or- flight response. Our heart rate increases, we breathe faster and our peripheral circulation increases to support our muscles. At the same time our central circulation decreases, digestion become slow and our immune response is compromised. When the acute stress phase is over, our body tries to return to normalcy by activating the Parasympathetic Nervous System (PNS). This put our body into **'rest and recovery'** or in **'growth' mode**. Our heart rate comes down to normalcy, breathing becomes slow and deep, digestion improves due to increased blood flow to internal organs and our immune response reactivate.

When we are in the protection for a longer period, our growth mechanism severely gets compromised and our immune response becomes slow. This immunosuppressive nature of stress makes us prone to diseases. Managing stress properly, strengthen our immunity. Meditation, affirmations, regular exercise and adequate sleep reduce stress and help our protector cells to grow.

Chapter XII

Care for Your Lifestyle

"Think and practice healthy rituals, health will follow. Health is your creation"
Author

"Lifestyle" is no more a simple word nowadays. It has been associated with almost every possible complication in this world. It is a great topic of discussion, from health and happiness to corporate and glamour world. Every patient I examine is a victim of the lifestyle diseases and every medical Seminar I attend discuss about implications of lifestyle on our health. Every health awareness program is about lifestyle diseases.

The moment I ask my patients to change their lifestyle, I see a big confusion on their face. The first question they ask me, "Doctor, can you explain to me what should I do?" I always used to answer in a stereotype way. Change your food habit, exercise daily, and reduce your stress etc. However, from deep down inside I am fully aware that, these simple monosyllables were not enough to change someone's lifestyle. We have to tell them in details and motivate them for a better life. This chapter is for understanding "what lifestyle is about and how to manage it".

Lifestyle is nothing but the interests, opinions, behaviours, and behavioural orientations of an individual, group or culture. It is the way or the style of living. It reflects our attitude, values and our views towards this world. Lifestyle includes our views on politics, religion, health, intimacy and more. Lifestyle is the way we cope with our physical, psychological, social and economical need on a day-to-day basis. It also reflects our self-image or self-confidence, which reflects the way we see ourselves and want to be seen by others. It is a combination of our needs and our motivation to achieve certain things.

"Care for your health" is all about promoting healthy lifestyle by empowering people with knowledge about their own body, so that they can take the necessary steps to keep themselves healthy. This book recommends changing lifestyle into this L.I.F.E.S.T.Y.L.E. way.

L - Learning, unlearning and relearning

I - Information and interpretations

F - Following our passions

E - Eating right and energising self.

S - Structuring our life

T - Training our body and Mind

Y - Yearning for a better I

L - Loving ourselves

E - Enjoying life

Learning, Unlearning and Relearning

Someone has rightly said, "To be knowledgeable, learn new things every day; to be wise, unlearn things that you have learnt with wit and love".

The same thing is applicable to our lifestyle. Our lifestyle is what we have learned during our lifetime from our immediate environment, from our parents and peers, from our education system and from the job, we do. We developed certain belief systems, which become an integral part of our life. We are constantly learning from our life's journey. Many times, we adopt certain beliefs and habits, which are not favourable to our health. The moment we realise this, it is the time to start identifying the factors responsible for our ill health. The next step should be to gradually, unlearn the things so that we will not repeat them. Once we are able to unlearn them, we should start relearning new things, which will help us to live a healthy life. It is unfortunate that we stop relearning or adopting new things after a certain age. It needs an open mindset to change our lifestyle for a better health.

Information and Interpretation

We are living in the information era, where all the information is at our fingertips. The problem is with the information *overload* and the fear of crossing the thin line, which separates information from misinformation. We have to constantly update our knowledge base regarding our health from the right source, and apply it in our life. Reading scientific journals, attending health seminars, talking to health professionals when we are healthy, and self help health books can enhance our knowledge about good health.

The most important thing is the way we interpret the information and apply it in our life. Interpretation is the act of explaining and reframing of the information. We have to customize information before applying it ourselves.

What is good for health to someone may not be good for me. The lifestyle changes should be very much individualized (varies from individual to individual).

Following Our Passion

Lifestyle is all about following our passion to fulfil our mission in life. When we are passionate about things we love, every cell from our body are in harmony with nature to keep us healthy. Passion is the desire to do something that a person likes to do or think is important to do. It brings us joy, happiness and a sense of fulfilment. Today's fast lifestyle has become a great obstacle to our passion. We all are in a rat race, where we want to compete with the person next to us, to show our supremacy. Our present lifestyle forces us to live, from 9 am to 5 pm, from Monday to Friday, in a hurry, with a stressed body and mind. Following the passion is becoming a rare phenomenon. Passion is a life skill, that helps bring vitality to our work, our family and to our body and mind. It is critical to our health. It compels us to go where we might not normally go.

The moment we change our lifestyle to follow our passion, we unblock many of the expressions we always wanted to express. It may be the job we hate or a relationship we want to get away. We can always revive the boundless energy within us by just following our passions. Our creativity and inspiration pulls us towards our passion.

Eating Right and Energizing Ourselves

All the lifestyle diseases are the product of our present eating habits. We are what our ancestors ate. There is a tremendous variation in what food; human can thrive on, depending on the genetic inheritance. Many studies have proved that, all these lifestyle problems started when we abandoned our traditional diet and active lifestyle. In the second half of the twentieth century, our diet changed dramatically; with the increased consumption of meat, dairy products, processed foods, vegetables oils and alcoholic beverages. There is a decreased consumption of fruits, vegetables, and high fibre and high water content food. This resulted in the increased burden of lifestyle disorders in the society.

If we follow the principles of food consumption as described in the Care for Your Food and fluid chapter, we will be able to reverse and prevent many of the lifestyle diseases. The basic principle remains to eat food available in the locality we are residing and go back to the high fibre and water and mineral rich foods.

Structuring Our Life

Structuring life is a way to organise our life in such a way that we can perform our best, effortlessly without much of a burden on self. Structuring life is nothing but planning for the next twenty-four hours beforehand. It creates stability and balance in our life. It is necessary for the people who want to bring a change in their lifestyle. Bringing structure into our life is like pouring water into a structured glass. If there is no structured thing like glass to hold the water, we cannot drink it. Exactly, if we do not bring all of our work into a structured form, it is impossible to give justice to our work.

Jim Rohn has said; "Either you run the day or the day runs you". Best way to start structuring our life is to follow certain routine in life and develop some good habits. Routines like getting up at a particular time, 30 to 45 minutes of exercise every day, a good breakfast, starting the day's work at a fixed time, separate time to meet clients etc can make a difference in our life.

Few tips for structuring life:

1. Let us start maintaining a planner and note down the future tasks as it comes to us.

2. Hourly planner to be filled, a night before keeping sufficient buffering time.

3. We should stick to the morning routine without fail. This creates a sense of perfection and accomplishment and boosts our morale for the whole day.

4. Eating time to be given priority and should be fixed at the same time every day.

5. Always we should create deadlines for every work we start.

6. For meditation and prayer, we should keep at least 30 minutes every day.

Training of Our Mind and Body

"Mind is the master of our body. If we train and discipline our mind, body will follow".

Robert Jones.

We should have a strong mind to bring changes in our lifestyle. We have to prepare ourselves mentally first by visualizing the end results. Stephen covey in his bestselling book, "The Seven Habits of Highly Effective People" mentions it as Habit II, 'Begin with the End in Mind'. The moment our mind is ready for a lifestyle change, our body will follow by materialising the plan. To train our mind our focus should be on what makes us happy.

Training our body is the way; we keep ourselves active and fit. When our body follows an exercise schedule, every cell tries to be in harmony with nature. Training our body is to make it healthy by taking care of it. This is possible by regular exercise and a balanced nutrition. The first thing to train our body is to have a training goal and put all our efforts to achieve it.

Yearning for a Better I

Yearning means a feeling of intense longing for something we do not have at present. Yearning for a great body, healthy organs, a peaceful mind, love, respect, status in the society is a part of our lifestyle. The more we climb the ladder of success, the more we go crazy. When the direction of our yearning turns towards a better us, things around us will change accordingly.

Yearning for a better you, starts with questioning self, what more I need to increase the happiness within me and around me? When we look for the answer, the whole universe becomes a guide and shows the path towards a better us.

When the yearning goes outward, giving becomes a part of our life rather than taking. We will be in a win-win situation forever. We become empathetic and sharing becomes a part of our life. This yearning will bring a **style in our life.**

Loving Ourselves

"Life is a voyage of self discovery. To me, to be enlightened is to go within and to know who and what we really are, and to know that we have the ability to change for the better by loving and taking care of ourselves ". Louise Hay.

We have been taught from the beginning of our life that 'Love is God'. Loving self is, loving the God within us. As we move forward in our life's journey, our love towards self diminishes and we start showing our love toward other, in an effort to make others happy. The society we live considers self-love as selfishness. Unfortunately, today's lifestyle keeps no space left for self-love. We go on exploiting ourselves for material and short-term gain. By the time we realise, it is too late.

When we love ourselves, we recognise our strength and our self-confidence level goes up. Self-love leads to self-care. When we take care of ourselves, we lead a healthy life. When we love ourselves, we will be motivated to change our lifestyle for a healthier us.

Enjoying Life

Enjoying life means doing things which we love to do at a particular point of time, without any external interference or influence. However, unfortunately our lifestyle forces us to enjoy our life with certain conditions attached. We give more importance to others opinion. Let us ask ourselves, am I doing the right thing? Am I excited about it? If the answer is no, then we are not enjoying life. The meaning of enjoying life varies from person to person and from time to time. Our lifestyle should allow us to get few moments of our life to spend, for the things we always want from the deepest core of our heart. All these are small things but matters a lot for the health and well-being of an individual. It is just giving priority to things that are really important to us, we start enjoying life. Few things we can do to enjoy life.

- Finding time to visit our near and dear ones,
- Going for a movie we wanted to see but missed it due to other engagements,
- Finding out time to relax and getting connected to self,
- Visiting new places and meeting people of different culture,
- Following our passion, experimenting on new things,
- Celebrating success,
- Creating a sanctuary around us,
- Sharing our thoughts and experiences with others,
- Learning new skills and
- Becoming a part of the changes happening around us.

Chapter XIII

Conclusion (The Summery)

'Using the amazing power of the human body, it is easier to maintain a sound body and mind forever than restoring normalcy from a diseased state. Start working on yourself, before you have a disease'.

Author

Care for your health is just a user manual to empower you with a basic understanding about the functioning of our body. God has sent us to this world healthy and it is our responsibility to keep ourselves healthy life long. Our body is a wonderful machine that comes with the self-correction buttons, which we are unaware off. This book provides all the information to find out those switches and use them judiciously to remain healthy throughout life. This book will convince you that there is no magic formula to health; it is only by sincerely following certain basic rituals to maintain our body and mind by which we will remain healthy. There are certain 'Must do', which we have to do every day. This is like taking the control in our hand.

The information provided in the "Care for your cells" chapter; empowers us with the basic understanding of the cellular health. We have all the power to keep our cells healthy till we die, if we can provide them with the right environment. Our thoughts and belief system play a major role. We have the power to program and reprogram our cells for a better life. We no longer believe that we are born with the predetermined fate, locked inside our genes. We can alter our genes on a regular basis depending on the environment we provide them. The food we eat, the air we breathe, and the thought we think becomes our environment, which dictates our health status. Therefore, at the epigenetic level, we have the power to alter the course of our diseased cells, by just changing our environmental parameters.

The chapter on 'care for your breath' provides us the information about the most important ingredient of life 'AIR'. Air is life but most of the time, most of the people sub optimally use the power of our breathing and the breathing apparatus. The basic instructions given, if followed, will enable you to lead a healthy life forever. Deep and conscious breathing technique through pranayama is a must for a healthy and disease free life.

Care for your heart provides the inside story of our heart and leaves a clear message that if we take care of our cholesterol and develop habits of exercise daily there is a chance that we will have a perfect heart health till death.

Care for our gut unfolds the role of our microbiota, which controls our biology to a great extent. The chapter establishes the fact that the gut is our second brain and it controls our behaviour through the 'Gut Brain Axis'.

Care for our mind tells us the role of mind over body. Our emotions and the behaviours directly affect us through the biologically active molecules present all over the body. We are now convinced that, we are 'body of minds' as the intelligent molecules present all over our body sends, analyses and receive information just like us. Stress is the biggest modern day enemy and this chapter provides a solution for the management of stress through S.T.R.E.S.S. Formula.

The care for your aging chapter tells us that age is just a number. If we can make a balance between the two biological processes, entropy and the homeostasis, then we can slow down our aging process.

Care for your bones and muscles gives emphasis on the importance of metabolically active muscle mass. We can remain strong and active until we die without any debilitating diseases, if we strengthen our muscle mass through resistance training. We can avoid osteoporosis by good nutrition and strength training.

Care for our food and fluids tell us about the importance of food in our life. This chapter busts many of the myths about food. It is the source of energy, if properly planned will keep us healthy for a longer period. The most important fluid is water, which is required for millions of chemical reactions happening in your body and is a wonderful transport medium because of its great dissolving capability.

Care for our protectors unveiled the power of our natural protective mechanisms present in our body. If we take care of them and help them to perform at their best, there is a hope for living a healthy life forever.

We all discuss about the present day lifestyle wherever we go. In reality, we never bother to apply it in our life, thinking it is not for me. The reason being, no one discusses about it in details with us. In the final chapter of, "Care for your lifestyle", we have discussed about it in details in L.I.F.E.S.T.Y.L.E way. Let us understand lifestyle, to apply it in our life.

Repetition, repetition and repetition is the principle of this book. We have repeated the five most important requirements of healthy living air, water, food, mind and exercise, many times in this book. We have to understand that, all of our systems and cells are interconnected and interdependent. Our cells and our organs follow the principle of cooperation. Taking care of one system boosts the efficiency of other system to some extent. Care for your health has put light on all the systems briefly, so that we can start working on our body to keep it healthy and remain vibrant forever.

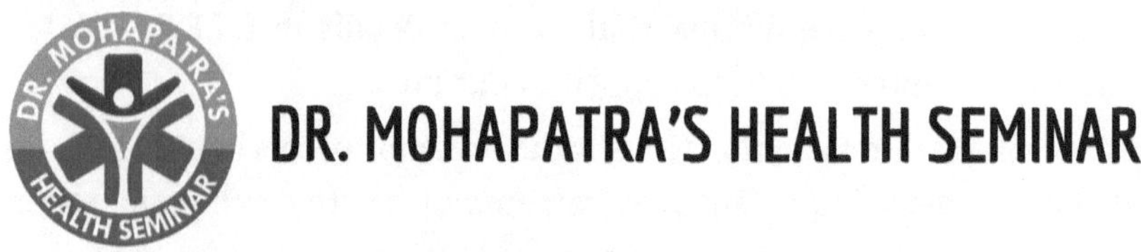

My Health is my Responsibility; let's discuss Health, No Disease Please.

Dear Readers,

Dr. Mohapatra's Health Seminar is a non medicalised health motivational seminar, where we discuss only about your health. Extraordinary healing stories, basic knowledge about your body, exercise physiology, truth about nutrition, power of your mind, **inspires, educates and entertains** you to lead a life of your dream. This program is a blend of awareness and motivation for living a healthy life. We clearly differentiate between health and diseases through this seminar.

We strongly believe that; 'when health comes first, rest of the things follows'. For further details please contact

Dr. Biswajit Mohapatra, MS

bmdoc1@gmail.com

9437042490

www.ingramcontent.com/pod-product-compliance
Lightning Source LLC
Chambersburg PA
CBHW031238250726
48655CB00005B/2004